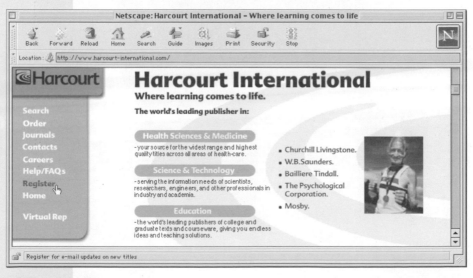

Promoting Men's Health

Neil Davidson has been involved in work with young and adult men for over 15 years, in particular focusing on sex education and sexual health. As co-director of the organisation Working With Men he has been involved in consultancy, training, research and speaking on issues concerning men's health for several years. His publications include: *Boys Will Be...? Sex Education And Young Men* (1991), *Vitality And Virility: Sexual Health For Mid-life Men* (1995), *Men's Sexual Health Matters* (1998). He is also co-editor of Working With Men's own magazine *WWM*. He is currently involved in a 2-year project developing work with young men on preventing teenage pregnancy.

Trefor Lloyd has been involved in developing work with men for over 17 years. He co-founded The B Team in 1985 to produce useful resources and publications for those developing work with men, and Working With Men to provide training and consultancy and a subscription journal to the same professionals. He has written and spoken in Britain and abroad on issues affecting men, but especially about the development of practice. Publications and research include: *Work With Boys* (1985); *Working With Men Who Batter their Partners* (with John Lees, 1993); *Young Men's Health: A Youthwork Concern* (1996); *What Next for Men?* (with Tristan Wood, 1996); *A Review of Men's Health Literature* for the RCN's Men's Health Forum (1996); *Let's Get Changed Lads: Developing Work With Boys and Young Men* (1997); *Running the Risk: young men's perceptions of risk-taking, health and local services in Birmingham* (1997); *Reading for the Future: Boys' and Fathers' Views on Reading* (1998); *Perceptions of Men: Young Children Talking* (with Save the Children, 1997); Briefing paper on public health implications on men's health for the Men's Health Forum (1998); Briefing paper on inequalities in health: implications on men's health (1999); *Young Men, the Job Market and Gendered Work* (Joseph Rowntree Foundation, York 1999); *Fatherhood Game and Pack* (a curriculum pack for schools) (1999); Health Education Authority *Directory of Resources on Men's Health* (with Neil Davidson, in press); policy paper on *Young Men and Suicide* for The Men's Health Forum (in press). Current projects include: A 3-year Home Office project developing community-based models of working with fathers, an information pack for young fathers and running support groups for new fathers; *Preparing young men for work* (funded by Joseph Rowntree Foundation) - this project involves the delivery of modules to year 10 boys at risk of exclusion.

For Baillière Tindall:

Senior Commissioning Editor: Sarena Wolfaard
Project Development Manager: Karen Gilmour
Head of Project Management: Ewan Halley
Designer: George Ajayi

Promoting Men's Health
A Guide for Practitioners

Edited by

Neil Davidson
Working With Men, London

Trefor Lloyd
Director, Working With Men, London

Foreword by

Ian Banks
Chairman, Royal College of Nursing Men's Health Forum

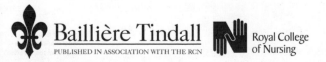

Baillière Tindall
PUBLISHED IN ASSOCIATION WITH THE RCN

Royal College
of Nursing

EDINBURGH LONDON NEW YORK PHILADELPHIA ST LOUIS SYDNEY TORONTO 2001

BAILLIÈRE TINDALL
An imprint of Harcourt Publishers Limited

© Harcourt Publishers Limited 2001

✤ is a registered trademark of Harcourt Publishers Limited

The right of Neil Davidson and Trefor Lloyd to be identified as editors of
this work has been asserted by them in accordance with the Copyright,
Designs and Patents Act 1988

First published 2001

ISBN 0 7020 2416 3

British Library Cataloguing in Publication Data
A catalogue record for this book is available from the British Library

Library of Congress Cataloging in Publication Data
A catalog record for this book is available from the Library of Congress

The
publisher's
policy is to use
paper manufactured
from sustainable forests

Printed in China

Contents

Contributors

Peter Baker
Was contributing health and fitness editor of *Maxim* magazine from 1995 to 1999 and writes extensively on men's health issues. He has been published regularly in the *Observer* and *Independent*, *Healthlines* and *Here's Health*. He is on the executive committees of The Guild of Health Writers and the Men's Health Forum, is co-author of *The MANual: The Complete Man's Guide to Life* (Thorsons, 1996) and author of *Total Well Man: A Complete Guide to Health and Well-being for Life* (Element, 2000).

Mina Bhavsar
Formerly health policy officer: equality and health, at Leicester City Council Unitary Authority. Now project manager of Project DIL, funded by the Department of Health and supported by Leicestershire Health Authority, with the aim of reducing coronary heart disease risk factors in the South Asian community.

Paul Brown
Chief executive of Leicester Young Men's Christian Association.

Christina Lynne Evans
Lecturer at HMYOI Deerbolt, and freelance researcher and consultant.

Richard Fletcher
Lecturer at the Family Action Centre, adjunct lecturer in the Faculty of Medicine and Health Sciences, and manager of the Men and Boys Program at the University of Newcastle, New South Wales, Australia.

Paul Flowers
Formerly of the MRC Social and Public Health Sciences Unit at the University of Glasgow. Now Lecturer in Health Psychology at Glasgow Caledonian University.

Siân Griffiths
Director of Public Health and Health Policy for Oxfordshire.

Lesley Hamilton
Locality health promotion specialist, Northamptonshire Health Authority.

David Hart
Community mental health nurse working for Community Health Sheffield Trust.

Graham Hart
Associate Director of the MRC Social and Public Health Sciences Unit at the University of Glasgow.

Lorraine Hoare
Health Education Authority.

David Jewell
Consultant senior lecturer in Primary Care, University of Bristol. Also a general practitioner for nearly 20 years. Editor of the *British Journal of General Practice*, and co-editor of *Men's Health*, a book for health professionals.

Alec Kendall
Assistant Director of Public Health, Worcestershire Health Authority.

Judi Keshet-Orr
Consultant psychosexual and relationship therapist at the Whittington Hospital NHS Trust. Course director for the Postgraduate Diploma and MSc in Psychotherapy and Psychosexual Therapy, Middlesex University and Whittington Hospital collaborative project. Also in private practice. Chair of BASNT Accreditation Board. Consultant and Supervisor in the UK and overseas.

Brian MacKenzie
Formerly director of Health Works, Dorset's Health Promotion Agency. Now consultant in Health and Community Development, Bournemouth University.

Mike Massaro
Project manager for the Health Opportunities Team, where he has developed, delivered and evaluated sexual health related groupwork with young people, especially young men.

Tony Mays
Mental health social worker working for Sheffield Family and
Community Services.

Lindsay Neil
Freelance consultant; social research and policy development for HIV
prevention and AIDS care, in the UK and internationally.

Maggie Robinson
Development officer at the CEDC Community Education
Development Centre, Coventry. CEDC is an educational trust that
aims to widen opportunities for learning.

Terri Roche
East Surrey Health Promotion Unit.

Maya Twardzicki
East Surrey Health Promotion Unit.

Joan Walsh
Contraceptive Education Service.

Christine Watson
Formerly consultant in Family Planning and Reproductive Health,
Optimum Health Services NHS Trust.

David Wilkins
Health promotion coordinator, Health Works, Dorset, and
lecturer/practitioner in Health Promotion, University of
Bournemouth.

Phil Williams
Founder member (with Sandie Williams) of WCT Phoneline for men
with cancer (formerly Mind over Matter).

Foreword

Men's health is a bit of a contradiction in terms. Tellingly, some statistics stand out, not least the tragic level of suicide amongst young men, which is currently four times that in women. Even life expectancy differs between men and women and is compounded by social class. Despite the well-recognised facts, there has been almost a conspiracy of silence about men's health amongst politicians and within the media. Times change and over the past few years men's health as an issue has become increasingly prominent, with numerous books, articles, magazines and even political action. When a minister for public health such as Yvette Cooper MP publicly acknowledges the inequalities in health that exist and the lack of resources dedicated to men's health, things can only get better. The explosion in the number of books reflects increasing awareness but, like men's health, they are not all equal, ranging from turgid, unreadable tomes to superb collections of data, examples of good practice and recommendations. Neil Davidson and Trefor Lloyd from Working With Men highlighted men's health before others had even recognised there was such a phenomenon. Their publications and work provide a bedrock on which others can act to address the often atrocious state of health suffered by men, especially those in lower income and ethnic minority groups. This book is an elegant, readable, well-researched addition to their already impressive list. If those in a position to bring about change were to read and act on such quality information, men and health would be more likely to be compatible, not a contradiction.

Ian Banks
Chairman, Men's Health Forum

Preface

Why do we need a book on men's health? Is it any different to any-body else's health? Why should we be 'promoting' it? This book examines these and related questions currently being asked by many health professionals and others working with men. Our main aim here is to provide some starting points to help find the answers.

Since the mid-1990s, there has been a dramatic growth of interest in men's health amongst the wider public. There has been a spate of media and Government attention focusing in one way or another on the 'problem of men', or on a perceived 'crisis in masculinity'. We have had waves of concern about absent or feckless fathers, under-achieving boys, the lack of positive male role models, and men as violent and abusive partners. Complementing this problem-based focus has been a commercially orientated targeting of men's health and lifestyle needs, through the growth of the 'new men's media'. Although the 'problem' of men generally – and of their health in particular – is not actually new, what we have now is a climate in which there is increasing potential for actually addressing the major issues.

The development of work geared towards men's health issues is still in its infancy, but interest amongst the public and health profes-sionals has been growing since 1993 when, in his annual report on public health, the then Chief Medical Officer Kenneth Calman called for action to target health messages on men. The current Government's approach to health – *Our healthier nation* – with its emphasis on the wider social and economic context, suggests there is a potential for the growth of work on men's health. Yet this may not be straightforward. Finding an appropriate strategic context for work with men (which includes policy, practice, resourcing and wider changes in attitudes and social norms) has proved difficult in the past. The new public health approach of this Government may raise as many questions as it answers.

Health professionals have recently been made more aware of men's health needs and the barriers men encounter when seeking services. The profile of these issues has been raised through conferences, training events, and the formation of professional networks and lobbying groups such as the Royal College of Nursing's Men's Health Forum. This book seeks to address the most pressing needs of the professionals who provide health-related services to men. It will be of value to health promotion specialists, GPs, practice nurses, GUM and family planning staff, occupational health professionals, health visitors, social workers, community health workers, teachers and youth workers. It will also be of use to policy makers, academics and researchers.

In Part 1 we provide basic factual and statistical information on men's health and associated trends. Interwoven with this we try to build an understanding of the socialisation process which informs men's health behaviour, beliefs and attitudes.

Part 2 consists of invited contributions from practitioners who have pioneered work with men on health issues. We asked them to summarise what they have learned about the opportunities and barriers involved. In order to build on the growing recognition of the importance of a more strategic approach in this field, we have also included contributions from those with a strategic overview of local, national and international developments.

Part 3 summarises the main themes emerging from Part 2 and uses these as the foundation for guidelines on how work on men's health can be pushed forward most productively.

Men's health is still relatively unexplored territory and in a climate of change and reorientation of priorities this may understandably inhibit health professionals from embracing the new. We hope this book will provide not only information and useful advice but, most of all, inspiration to help practitioners, policy makers and managers to initiate work on men's health.

London, 2000   Neil Davidson and Trefor Lloyd

Acknowledgements

The editors would like to express their grateful appreciation to all the contributors for their hard work and patience.

... ...

Part 1

Men and health: the context for practice

This part covers:

- Men and health: the context for practice
- Inequalities in men's health
- Commissioning and men: the case of STDs.

In Part 1 we provide some statistical information on men's health and associated trends, and build an understanding of the socialisation process which informs men's health behaviour, beliefs and attitudes. We also examine how the commissioning process works in the NHS, as this influences greatly the sort of health promotion work that can be carried out.

1

Men and health: the context for practice

Trefor Lloyd

This chapter covers:

- what is men's health?
- the current context
- the new public health
- implications for men's health
- the broader context
- men's role and health
- what are the causes of men's poor health?
- masculinity in perspective
- gender role
- social relations
- cultural perspective
- feminism
- attitudes to health
- men's health behaviours
- the consequences for practice
- men's health services
- male suicide.

Introduction

It was the Chief Medical Officer's (CMO's) Annual Report for 1992 that detailed mortality and morbidity data for men and invited 'Regions and Districts to investigate ways to promote the health of men' (Calman 1993). The CMO highlighted coronary heart disease, cancers, sexual health, accidents, suicide and mental health as areas of particular concern for men and stated that 'although some diseases, such as prostatism, are obviously unique to men, the main differences in mortality and morbidity relate to variations in exposure to risk factors'. Although some men's health initiatives did exist before 1992, the CMO's report detailed the epidemiological evidence for the first time and encouraged us all to look more specifically at the behaviours and attitudes of men towards their health.

While the report has inspired a number of initiatives, our experience shows that there are still many professionals whose attitude can be summed up as follows: we are open to everyone; if men don't want to use the service, what can we do? In 1995, at a national conference on Men's Health Matters, one of the speakers involved in an ongoing population study began his talk with the comment that before he had been asked to make this presentation, he hadn't really considered the fact that his sample were all men. Honest – but also a reflection of the importance of focusing on men's health. In 1993, while carrying out a review of the way a national health promotion agency targeted men, we met with a number of senior managers who told us how bemused they were that we wanted to talk to them, explaining that if we wanted to talk about men's health, then we should move swiftly to the sexual health team. Some professionals (not only in primary healthcare) consider their (and their patients') gender to be of little importance. In their view they are professionals, are seen by their patients as genderless, and deal with males and females in the same way. Other people are more aware of the biological, predetermined differences between the sexes. Others feel quite simply that men will be men and women will be women – so what's the issue? There are those that think that primary healthcare services are already so severely stretched that more men using them would stretch them to breaking point. There is also a view that focusing on women's health is a distraction and a bit too political, so why would we want to walk down the same path with men's health? On the other hand, some feel that women's health has made (especially in primary healthcare) services lopsided, and we need to put resources into men's health to redress the balance. And of course there are those who think the issue of men's health is much too complex or contentious, or that there are more important needs to be met, or that it's not worth the risk (or the effort) of getting involved.

These, then, are some of the reasons that men's health needs to be addressed. Gender blindness, fear of having to deal with men, reluctance to acknowledge social factors in gender conditions and seeing gender as only biological – all these attitudes create barriers to providing a good service to male patients, especially within primary healthcare. But, as we know, health services (and especially primary healthcare) have been through almost constant change since 1993: introduction of the internal market; the abolition of Regional Health Authorities; the running down of health promotion services; the change of Government; the public health agenda; the dissolving of the internal market .... These have certainly been enough to distract health workers from any new initiatives, especially ones which pose many questions.

It is not our intention in this chapter to answer all of the questions. Instead, we will cover much of the ground these questions and perspectives highlight. We will examine some of the epidemiological evidence and research about particular conditions and health behaviours of men. We will look at the broader context of masculinity and detail emerging questions and priorities, and offer a framework in which to address men's health issues.

What is men's health?

There is a range of different models and definitions of health. Some stress inheritance, others socioeconomic circumstances, or behaviour and beliefs as being of primary importance. These differing models have influenced the way that men's health has been viewed. A 1996 review of men's health literature (Lloyd 1996) identified three prominent definitions:

1. Men's health is *biological* – e.g. prostate and testicular cancers, STDs and other sexual health matters.
2. Men's health is about *risk* and risk-taking.
3. Men's health is primarily about *masculinity* (the process of learning to be a man), and the impact this process has on the way men perceive their health.

The CMO's report showed that the primary difference between men's and women's health was 'variations in exposure to risk factors' (Calman 1993). The risk-taking definition sits within a lifestyle view of health, where individual men take risks and the health promotion task is to encourage them to stop. The biological is seen as important, the social is acknowledged, but fundamentally this model is concerned with an *individual's framework of beliefs and behaviours*. Where socialisation of men (masculinity) is acknowledged as a factor, it is often seen as an inadequate model, on the grounds that men are not a homogenous group. The common view is that if we target those that take the risk, then we will reach men. This means we need to know about the risk factors and not necessarily the people who take them.

Within the masculinity model, there are those who see masculinity as being of primary importance to men's health, while others identify social factors such as class, poverty, race and sexuality as being equally important. Some use masculinity as a unitary experience for men – 'Men can't express their feelings, separate their heads from their bodies' – while others discuss multiple masculinities, focusing as much on the differences between groups of men, as on the similarities.

The three main definitions outlined here inevitably reflect different perspectives on the broader question of what health is. It is unlikely that you will have a view that men's health is defined by masculinity and social factors *and* believe that health is primarily defined by biology; or that men's health is primarily biological *and* that health is determined by levels of personal risk factors. You may though, believe that health is influenced by a combination of biology, personal choice and social factors.

The point being made here is that definitions of men's health (like other health categories) are context specific and determined by wider belief systems and practice. Fletcher (who has written Chapter 5 of this book) takes this further. In an Australian report on men's health services compiled in 1997 he suggests that:

> In a very practical sense, men's health will be defined by whatever health workers say it is. If nurses demonstrating testicular self examination say they are doing 'Men's Health' then that is what will be associated with the name. If social workers running

programs for perpetrators of domestic violence say they are involved in 'Men's Health' then this activity will come under the banner too.

However, unless we define what men's health is, and clarify whether men's health is social, psychological, biological, individual, or all of these and more, then misunderstandings and a lopsided literature will continue, as will narrow strategies and developments. One-dimensional strategies have already followed from these partial definitions. Some have seen targeting as the major objective in men's health, others have identified the need for services specifically for men (Well Men clinics, for example), while others still have advocated concentrating on screening symptoms and other preventative measures. Clarity about how we define men's health is of central importance to any developing practice and services.

Fletcher has adapted the United States Public Health Service definition of women's health to come up with a useful working definition (see Ch. 5):

> A men's health issue is a disease or condition unique to men, more prevalent in men, more serious among men, for which risk factors are different for men or for which different interventions are required for men.

This is of course an inclusive definition, but it helps to contain a range of conditions, factors, groups of men and interventions which need to be considered by practitioners developing initiatives within a men's health framework.

How might a men's health movement develop? A MORI survey of District Directors of Public Health commissioned in 1995 by the RCN revealed concerns that a men's health movement might parallel the women's health movement. Some argue that this is not likely. Orr (1987) has suggested that the women's health movement developed in two ways: 'a medical model with emphasis on screening and physical health, usually initiated by professionals, and a holistic, self-health model evolving primarily out of the women's movement'. Robertson (1995) suggests this is most unlikely to happen in men's health, as the men's movement is not developed in the same way and men are not clamouring for services.

We would agree with this view, and suggest that women's health be used as a model to develop men's health only with some caution. For example, screening for breast cancer has been a very important women's health initiative. To translate this into screening for prostate cancer for men without acknowledging the differences in effectiveness of the screening process, the differences in the demands of men and women thought to be at risk and the settings that these services may be offered (and taken up) in would be too simplistic. There will be some similarities, but even these cannot be assumed.

The current context

A definition of men's health will also need to be adaptable, dependent on the context of the health model being used. The CMO's report for 1992 was written within the context of an individual framework of beliefs and behaviours. The Government was in the process of shifting the focus of the NHS from treating sickness towards promoting health by emphasising the individual's capacity to change behaviour (Calman 1993). The current Labour Government wants to take this still further. Its 1998 Green Paper, *Our healthier nation*, stated:

> setting out the case for concerted action to tackle not just the causes of disease but the causes of the causes: poverty, inequalities, social exclusion, unemployment, and the other features of the physical and social environment that converge to undermine health. (Department of Health 1998b)

The rationale for this change in emphasis was that:

> the link between poverty and ill health is clear. In nearly every case the highest incidence of illness is experienced by the worst off social classes ... Individuals on their own find it hard to make a difference. But with help from their families and support, when needed, from the community and local agencies they can make real changes. Local agencies need central Government to provide leadership and put in place the national building blocks and support. Without individuals, families and communities working together, Government achievements will be limited ... In the past, arguments about health ranged between two extremes – individual victim blaming on the one hand and nanny state social engineering on the other. The broad majority who just wanted a normal healthy life for themselves and their families were ignored. (ibid.)

The new public health

Since the Government's health strategy was announced in July 1997, there has been considerable debate about what the 'new public health' agenda is and how it might operate. Concerns about whether the public health model is up to a new role have been raised – 'an old vehicle was being driven into a new era' (Warden 1998). Much of the debate has focused on where, when and how rather than what. Whether public health should be within health authorities, or local authorities (see e.g. Clarke, Hunter & Wistow 1997), whether the depleted local government infrastructures were up to the new role, or whether the consultant-orientated health services could refocus to a public health agenda, whether social, rather than medical models of health could be incorporated and whether health and local authorities are able and willing to enter into a public health partnership (Cohen 1998a, 1998b).

The Government's view appears to reflect what Ashton & Seymour (1988) have called the New Public Health which:

> goes beyond an understanding of human biology and recognises the importance of those social aspects of health problems which are caused by life-styles. In this way it seeks to avoid the trap of blaming the victim. Many contemporary health problems are therefore seen as being social rather than solely individual problems; underlying them are concrete issues of local and national public policy, and what are needed to address these problems are 'Healthy Public Policies' – policies in many fields which support the promotion of health. In the New Public Health the environment is social and psychological as well as physical.

Implications for men's health

Current definitions of men's health will have to incorporate these contextual changes. Men's health is to be seen as being affected by social, psychological, biological as well as physical factors. Conditions, attitudes and behaviours are to be understood in the context of the social and psychological aspects of masculinity. This will also involve taking into account other issues that make up the broader context of men's health. Individual risk-taking is of enormous importance; but so are a man losing his job, the messages he received about growing up to be a man (and how much he feels the need to prove this), where he lives, and with whom.

The broader context

Having suggested a definition for men's health and described the public health context in which men's health needs to be understood, we can now move on to what we do and don't know in terms of statistical and epidemiological evidence.

A public health approach requires men's health to be seen in a much wider context of changes affecting men and the way that these changes also affect others. To illustrate this wider context, some of the trends that are particularly male-specific are detailed below. (For detailed mortality and morbidity figures and specific conditions see O'Dowd & Jewell 1998 and Drever & Whitehead 1997.)

- *Male morbidity exceeds female morbidity from conception throughout the lifespan.* The most generally accepted figure is that 120–160 males are conceived for every 100 females, with the sex differential having dropped to approximately 106:100 by birth (Ounsted 1972).

- *Men die younger than women.* Life expectancy in the UK for those born in 1996 is 79.7 years for women and 74.7 years for men. Throughout the 20th century, there was at least 5 years' difference between men and women. A similar difference exists in other EU countries (Department of Health 1992).

- *Causes of male deaths vary significantly with age*

  15–34 years

  - 21% road vehicle accidents
  - 20% other causes of injury and poisoning
  - 17% suicide

  35–54 years

  - 28% heart disease
  - 17% cancers
  - 12% suicide, injury and poisoning

55–74 years

– 34% heart disease
– 23% cancers

(OPCS 1992)

■ *These causes of death are similar to those of other European countries.* Circulatory disease, cancers and external injuries and poisoning account for about 80% of deaths in UK men under 65 years and 70–80% in other EU countries (Calman 1993).

■ *There are significant social class differences in most of these causes of male deaths.*

There is a four-fold difference in morality from accidents and from suicide and undetermined injury between the top and the bottom of the social class scale. For lung cancer, the differential is even greater, nearly five-fold. For stroke and ischaemic heart disease, class V has three times the mortality of class I and the other classes, class V having twice the SMR of class IV for these causes of death. For stroke, ischaemic heart disease and lung cancer, the gap between class V and the other classes is still considerable (Drever & Whitehead 1997).

■ *Accidents accounted for 1.9% of all deaths in 1991, but were the cause of 42% of all deaths of 15–24-year-old men, and 17% of 25–44-year-old men.*

Road traffic accidents are the single largest cause of accidental death in young people. Risk-taking behaviour, combined with lack of experience, alcohol and, to a lesser extent, drugs, are significant factors in accident causation for this age group (HMSO 1991). 49% of male accidental deaths in 1991 in those under 15 were caused by motor vehicle traffic accidents. In addition, an estimated 10 000 children a year are left with long-term health problems resulting from accidents.

■ *Suicide is four times more common in men than in women.* While women's suicide rates have been steadily decreasing since the mid-1970s, there has been a corresponding increase in men's rates – especially amongst young men. Men from social classes I and V are most likely to commit suicide. Unemployed men have two to three times the suicide rate of those in employment; single, divorced and widowed men have three times the rate of men with partners; and men with

AIDS, men in prison or abusers of alcohol and drugs are also at higher risk of suicide (Charlton et al 1993).

Male mortality and morbidity are examined in Chapter 2. (For detailed information on specific conditions see O'Dowd & Jewell 1998 and Drever & Whitehead 1997.) The strongest conclusion to be drawn from the morbidity data is that social class and age must be taken into account when looking at men's health. However, there are a number of other indicators which also have a bearing on men's health, and which suggest that dramatic changes have been going on in many men's lives since the late 1970s. Some of these are examined below.

- *Men are no longer primary breadwinners.* Britain is the first EU country to have a workforce consisting of more women than men. From 1979 to 1994 there was a 16.8% drop in the number of men in employment and a 12.2% increase in the number of women (OPCS 1994). Researchers monitoring these changes have estimated that 90% of the jobs created in this period have been perceived as being 'women's work' (i.e. with low pay, part-time, requiring small fingers), while a similar percentage of jobs lost were seen as 'men's jobs' (i.e. full-time, with wages high enough to keep a family, particularly manual or skilled labour) (HMSO 1993).

- *Unemployment rates for younger men have continued to rise.* (see Table 1.1). Young men experience more long-term unemployment. In 1997, 18–24-year-old males who had been unemployed for over a year outnumbered females by more than 3:1. And the longer the period of unemployment, the wider the gap between men and women becomes (Department of Employment 1997)

- *The more unskilled a man is, the more likely he is to be unemployed.* According to a Labour Party analysis of official

Table 1.1   **Unemployment rates (%) for young men (after Department of Employment 1997)**

Age	1991	1996
16–19	16.4	20.6
20–24	15.2	16.2

figures (Burghes, Clarke & Cronin 1997), up to 40% of men without qualifications are out of work, and the numbers are growing.

■ *The unemployment rate for black and Asian men is even higher.* Whether compared with white men or with black and Asian women. Figures from 1997 show the unemployment rate for white men to be 8% (white women 5%), compared to African-Caribbean and African men at 21% (women 14%), Indian men 10% (women 7%) and Pakistani and Bangladeshi men 18% (women 7%) (Department of Employment 1997).

Certain groups of men have been particularly badly affected by these changes.

■ young men under 25, and men over 50
■ men from social classes IV and V
■ those from areas where industrial and manufacturing industries were by far the major employers (such as the docks in the North East and Merseyside, mining in Yorkshire and South Wales and the car industries of the Midlands)
■ African-Caribbean and Bangladeshi men in particular, and black men generally
■ disabled men
■ men who have mental illness and/or criminal records (Department of Employment 1997).

The loss of well-paid and high-status jobs, particularly in manufacturing and heavy industries, has inevitably had a knock-on effect on many families, and is thought to have contributed to increased divorce rates and the break-up of families (Burgess & Ruxton 1996, Burghes, Clarke & Cronin 1997) These are not the only changes in men's lives though, as is shown below.

■ *The loss of social networks.* Many men's social networks are linked with their work. They socialise through and after work. For such men, where there is no work, there are no networks. Research has suggested that social exclusion is a major component of the psychological isolation that unemployed men experience (Kilmartin 1994).

■ *Crime continues to be a male preserve.* 96% of the prison population in England and Wales in 1996 was male (41 323 men compared to 1732 women). Of those found guilty of offences, 87.6% were male, 73.5% of those cautioned were male, as were 87.7% of those sentenced for indictable offences (Home Office 1994a, 1997). The majority of victims of violent crime are male (67% in 1990), at least 43% of whom were victims of either pub or street brawls. 32% of females were victims of domestic violence (Government Statistical Service 1990).

■ *Sexual offences have increased.* Notifiable sexual offences in England and Wales rose from 21 107 in 1980 to 29 044 in 1990. Of these, rape rose from 1225 to 3391 incidents; indecent assault on a female from 11 498 to 15 783; indecent assault on a male from 2288 to 3430 (Home Office 1994a, 1997).

■ *Male drug addiction is rising.* The number of male drug addicts notified to the Home Office went up three-fold from 2979 in 1983 to 8981 in 1993. The number of male 21–30-year-olds increased by 1562 to 5058. Figures from this time showed that males accounted for 77.7% of all addicts; 72% of these were under 30 years old (Home Office 1994b).

■ *Academic achievement is becoming a female preserve.* The underachievement of boys in education is of concern to educationalists, young men and parents alike. In 1993, 45.8% of girls gained five top grade GCSEs (grades A, B, or C), compared with only 36.8% of boys. And 16% of girls gained three or more A levels, compared to 14% of boys. Women made up 53% of the university population: 45.4% of women graduates were in work within 6 months of leaving university, as opposed to 42.3% of men. A year after graduating, 12% of men were unemployed, but only 8% of women (*The Sunday Times* 1994).

Boys have more problems at school. Research from Keele University in 1994 showed that up to 12% of boys aged 11–16 were unhappy and disillusioned at school (double the proportion of girls). Boys were also twice as likely to truant, do no homework and misbehave in lessons. Boys outnumber girls by 2:1 in Britain's schools for children with learning difficulties. In special units for behavioural problems, there are six boys for every girl (*The Sunday Times* 1998, Department of Education 1993). A MORI poll of 79 local authorities conducted in 1993 showed that African-Caribbean boys were four times more likely to be excluded from school than white boys. African–Caribbean children represented 8.1% of all children excluded though they made up only 2% of the school population.

Men's loss of traditional work (especially in social classes IV and V) has been linked with boys' underachievement at school (Bray et al 1997), with high levels of crime (*The Sunday Times* 1994), and with the increase in reported violence towards women and children (Burgess & Ruxton 1996, Burghes, Clarke & Cronin 1997). It has also led to raised expectations about men's domestic participation as fathers. Parallel with these have come the demands of the Child Support Agency, and debates about whether men's role in their children's lives should be merely financial (Dench 1996).

Men's role and health

The difficulties that the changes outlined above have created have been compounded by men's (and women's) narrow view of what it is to be a 'man', which focuses mainly on being a provider and protector, and being strong in mind and body. Both men and women have become uncertain about gender roles in contemporary society. The media discusses whether men are 'redundant'; some men find extreme ways to show that they are still 'real' men; there are increasing divorce and rela-tionship difficulties, and concerns about how boys are growing up and who their role models are; suicide rates among young men are rising (Lloyd 1997).

Men's behaviours and the effects of these changes on them are central to their health. For example, the experience of unemployment has been shown to destroy men's personal and social identities (especially their 'breadwinner' identity), often resulting in a life crisis, with the inevitable increase in stress and illness. The loss of income affects diet and other basic needs. Long-standing illness is 40% higher amongst unemployed men than men in work. It has been shown that the deterioration in men's mental health when they are unemployed improves if they return to work (Brenner 1979, Lewis 1998).

It is important to recognise at this point that we have a data problem. As mentioned above, the CMO's report (Calman 1993) provided a jolt in our awareness of men's health, and an invitation to look at the existing data in a way that few had done before. Kimmel (1994) has suggested that men and masculinity have been invisible, that it has taken women questioning femininity and gender for us to finally address what it means to be a man and what impact this has on men's lives and health. An obvious effect of this 'invisibility' is that researchers have not been asking the questions that we now need answers to. In such an evidence-led sector as health, we are lacking substantive research and findings, especially in such crucial cause-and-effect areas as:

- what is the impact of the loss of the traditional role on men's health?
- how much are accidents a result of young men trying to prove they are men?
- how do we know whether focusing on masculinity will result in saving men's lives?

This has often led us to rely on morbidity and mortality data, because it is 'hard evidence', along with employment, crime and educational attainment statistics. Because we stay with what's 'hard', that which we can point to as 'truth', we are limited in our ability to develop potentially more effective practice. All the while we are in danger of getting stuck in a vicious circle: we don't have the evidence, so we can't act; we can't give the resources to getting the evidence, because we don't know whether it is worth putting them there; we won't know that unless we have the evidence.

What are the causes of men's poor health?

There is evidence to show that biology plays a part in the gender differences in mortality:

- women are thought to have consistently lower neuro-endocrine and cardiovascular reactivity to stressors than men (Manuk & Polefrone 1987)
- men are thought to have a life-long sensitivity to certain prostaglandin metabolites that put them at higher risk of vascular damage and coronary disease then women (Ramsey & Ramwell 1984)

- at a general level, it is believed that genetic differences protect women from certain genetic diseases, and hormonal differences make men vulnerable to some diseases while protecting women (Kilmartin 1994).

However, it is generally accepted that these biological differences do not account wholly for the difference in mortality rates. Some studies have suggested that biological protection can be removed by behavioural factors. Templer, Griffin & Hintze (1993) have suggested that alcohol misuse accounts for an appreciable amount of the male life years lost, while Waldron (1988) posited that half of the mortality sex difference can be attributed to smoking. Reddy, Fleming & Adesso (1992) concluded that gender differentials in health were less a result of genetic factors and more due to conformance to behaviour socially defined as appropriate for men and women.

Verbrugge (1985), who remains one of the most influential writers in the field, ranks the factors that influence the gender differences in health. Most important, he suggests, are the acquired risks resulting from gender differences in roles, lifestyle, stress and preventative health practices. Next in importance are the differences in the perception and evaluation of illness, and the resulting action taken. Research has shown that the male gender role leads men to ignore their health needs.

Verbrugge (1985) for example explains the higher mortality rates for men as being:

> the outcome of differential risks acquired from role, stress, lifestyle, and preventative health practices. Psycho-social factors – how men and women perceive and evaluate symptoms, and their readiness and ability to take therapeutic action.

A number of studies have demonstrated a positive relationship between psychological masculinity and measures of mental health (e.g. Lewis 1988, Brenner 1979). Others have focused on more 'negative' aspects, such as emotional inexpression (Long 1989), and have found a strong correlation with mental health problems. Men who take on behaviour thought to be 'feminine' are thought by others to be 'less than men', whether it is because of 'self-disclosure' (Haviland 1988) or holding 'female' jobs, such as nursing (Derlega, Winstead & Jones 1991). This can lead to lower self-esteem and gender-role conflict and strain (Fitzgerald & Cherpas 1985), which becomes more of an issue if men are forced to take those jobs they perceive to be 'women's work'. 'Gender-role conflict is a negative psychological state that results from the contradictory and/or unrealistic demands of the gender role' (O'Neil 1990). Davis & Walsh (1988) found that there was a strong association between gender-role conflict and both low self-esteem and anxiety.

Reviewing biological, psychological and social factors, Kilmartin (1994) concluded that:

> males experienced a disproportionate number of childhood disorders, for example, attention deficit hyperactivity disorder and conduct disorder. Males constitute a majority of substance abusers, sexual deviants and people with behaviour-control problems such as pyromania, compulsive gambling, and angry outbursts. More men than women are diagnosed as paranoid, antisocial, narcissistic and schizoid, and, of course, men are more likely to commit suicide.

Masculinity in perspective

So, is becoming a man harmful to your health? The answer is: maybe. As late as the 1960s masculinity and femininity were seen as separate and opposite. Attributes were assigned to one or the other. So, for example, men were strong and women emotional. With over 90% of men in full-time jobs, often with high enough wages to keep a family, masculinity was problematic only when individuals found themselves at the 'wrong' end of the spectrum (women showing masculine characteristics, for example). Such people were seen as needing help in developing sex-appropriate characteristics. This view of individuals' inability to 'fit in the right hole' is now seen as being conservative.

Gender role

The 1970s saw gender role theorists questioning this bipolar approach, and developing instead the androgyny model that saw a healthy identity as a combination of both feminine and masculine characteristics (Bem 1987). Androgyny suggested that traditional masculinity (seen as high in masculine and low in feminine attributes) was in fact problematic. This contributed to the questioning of sex-role stereotyping and to the move away from individuals being seen as needing to be taught and helped to develop 'appropriate' gender characteristics.

The 1980s saw the development of the gender role strain model, which confirmed the problematic nature of masculinity and femininity as raised by the androgyny model (and by feminism), but went on to suggest that wider changes in society (e.g. employment trends, women's higher expectations, the absence of war) had made it increasingly difficult (and inappropriate) for men and women to take on the attributes and behaviours thought previously to be appropriate to them. Therefore, rather than seeing the individuals as being inadequate in some way, the role strain model emphasised the mismatch between the individual and societal changes and expectations. Role strain advocates such as Pleck (1981) stressed the damage that this process had on individual men, as they tried to fit themselves into the male stereotype, and the mental health problems that being unemotional, and trying to prove themselves as men could have on them.

It is the role strain model that has most influenced men's health advocacy and the public health framework. According to this model, neither the individual nor the State is entirely to blame: the finger is pointed at the tensions between individual men and what they perceived as society's expectations of them as men, and their own perceptions of what a man is.

The literature examining these roles and expectations is fairly extensive. Studies of mother–infant interaction show differences in the treatment of boys and girls (even medical personnel have been found to treat them differently). Hanson (1984) found that new-born males were often described as being 'sturdy', 'handsome' or 'tough', while females were 'dainty', 'sweet', or 'charming', in spite of there being no differences in size or weight.

Early gender learning is thought to be unconscious, the result of males and females speaking, handling and treating boys and girls differently. By the age of 2, children are thought to have a partial understanding of what gender is, knowing whether they are a 'boy' or a 'girl'. Toys, picture books and television have all been found to distinguish between males and females (Giddens 1993). Books have been found to not only distinguish between males and females, but also to over-represent boys. Lenore Weitzman (1972) found that male and female activities differed, and that males played a much larger part in the stories and pictures than females – by a ratio of 11:1.

When animals with gender identities were included, the ratio was 95:1.

By the time children start school, they are thought to have a clear consciousness of gender differences, and boys and girls are often still encouraged to concentrate on different activities and sports. Peer groups are thought to play a major part in reinforcing and further shaping gender identity throughout a child's school career, with friendship circles both in and out of school often either all-boy or all-girl (Giddens 1993).

Another useful conceptual framework for practitioners has been the identification by role theorists of a set of 'social scripts' (such as the need for soldiers to defend society) that individuals are tailored to fit:

> Masculine roles involve a set of expectations for task-orientated behaviours that emphasises logic and rationality and de-emphasises emotional experience. From early childhood, boys come to value masculine traits and behaviours and devalue feminine ones. (Kilmartin 1994)

In the field of men's health this may help us to understand some of the factors that contribute to men's poor use of services. If men are 'taught' to be strong, not to complain, not to be wimps, then this will make it harder for them to go to their GP, because they will perceive this as being weak, whinging and wimpy.

Social relations

Another perspective sees masculinity as a set of distinctive practices which take their shape from social structures. Men are moulded by their inter-relationship with these structures. One of the main differences between gender role theory and this social relations perspective has been highlighted by writers such as Connell (1995), who has questioned the inevitability of gender role theory (which suggests that men will learn what they are told, passively). Connell suggests that the interplay between men and social structures is in fact about benefits and gains that individual men may get by accepting these roles and in some cases striving for the status and power that accompanies them. Some men, for example, will take such risks as driving fast and drinking too much, because the benefits and status attached to these risks (with their mates) may outweigh the risks to their health.

The social relations perspective leans heavily on gender role theory as the means of learning to be a man, but it also contributes a lot to discussions about motivation and the inter-related nature of masculinity, femininity and power.

Cultural perspective

The cultural perspective suggests that masculinity is transmitted from one generation to the next, although again the assumption is that this is learnt and that it is comprised of individuals' perception of themselves as well as of society and others. This perspective leans heavily on an understanding of culture that is 'passed down from generation to generation, through which ordinary people conduct and make sense of their everyday lives' (Edley & Wetherell 1995).

Cultural codes, visual images, historical changes and ideology are held to be important in this perspective, and learning is thought to take place through observation, others' actions, conscious and unconscious understandings and recognition of 'recycled culture'. Writers such as Gilmore (1990) see masculinity as a direct response to particular social and environmental conditions. He details a number of examples of situations where men are 'encouraged' to exhibit masculine qualities for their own (and others') survival. Klein has explored the relationship between masculinity and muscle, embodied in heroes such as Arnold Schwarzenegger and Sylvester Stallone. He believes bodybuilders sacrifice their health through the use of steroids 'in pursuit of ideal masculinity' (Klein 1995).

Feminism

The last important perspective to consider is that of critical feminism, which is:

> built on the premise that social inequality and power struggles profoundly inform gender relations and health outcomes. In addition to sex role theory's focus on gender identity, socialisation, and conformity to role expectations, critical feminist thinkers emphasise the power differences that suffuse relational processes between men and women, women and women, and men and men. (Klein 1995)

Some groups of men have tried to offer certain men's health issues as examples of what they believe is a feminist conspiracy against them, claiming that it is men who are now discriminated against (Farrell 1994). They cite the difference between the way the health services deal with breast cancer (and screening) and prostate cancer (and screening). Also the dramatic rise in male suicides. Farad (1994) amongst others, appears to be using men's health as a tool for peddling an antifeminist and sometimes an antiwomen line.

Some have responded to this view by arguing that:

> Many of the role expectations and psychological traits attached to masculinity in the current gender order, such as aggressiveness, ambition, success striving, virility, asceticism, and competitiveness are intricately tied to men's preoccupations with power over others and attempts to impose their definition of reality on others. (Farrell 1994)

This tension between feminism and other perspectives again leaves its mark on our approach to men's health. Whether we like to think about it or not, we are usually sympathetic towards our patients; we believe their suffering needs to be eased and alleviated where possible. On the whole, we don't blame patients for the actions they have taken – so smokers are generally treated the same as nonsmokers. We can even see them as victims. Some health professionals, however, do find it harder to feel sympathy towards male patients, especially if they fail to attend surgery early enough to be able to treat an illness effectively, or are not able to voice their symptoms in the alloted consultation time, or do not demonstrate gratitude for the treatment they receive.

Attitudes to health

The varied perspectives described above all shed light on important components of the impact masculinity has on men's attitudes and behaviours. But what can we say with some confidence about the impact these processes have on men's health behaviours? Research has shown that:

- Men and women have similar concepts of health, both seeing men as being healthier.

- Men stress being fit, strong, energetic, physically active and being in control, while women stress not being ill and never seeing a doctor (Saltonstall 1993).

- Men are more likely to talk about their bodies as machines, e.g. describing the heart as 'a pump', and tend to see exercise as more important than food and rest, while women tend to see food, rest, and then exercise, as important (Blaxter 1990).

- Middle-aged women have been reported as placing a greater value on health than middle-aged men (Lau et al 1986).

- Some men, who have memories of a younger 'naturally healthy' body, while interacting with masculine attitudinal and behavioural norms, construct a self-image or personal fable which sustains the individual's identity as a normal, healthy guy (Watson 1993).

- While men may suffer more disease, they are not permitted to be as expressive as women in their illness behaviour (Robertson 1995).

- In an effort to achieve masculine status and conform to the socially prescribed male role, men frequently engage in compensatory, aggressive, risk-taking behaviours which may predispose them to illness, injury, and even death.

- Explanations for the higher mortality rates for men have included differences in risk-taking (Wingard 1984).

In a study looking at common cold symptoms, men were found to be more likely to report symptoms, although a complex picture emerged, in which men reported only symptoms that were thought to leave their 'male image' intact. In addition, professionals tended to react differently to men's and women's symptoms – men were perceived as being less ill, while women were perceived as exaggerating illness (Macintyre 1990).

Men's health behaviours

Men's attitudes and behaviours are reflected in the way they use health services:

- men appear to leave intervention until later
- fewer men go to visit their GP
- those men that do go to their GP go less often than women (in 1990, for instance, for every visit a man made, a woman made 2.1 – 67 million visits versus 143 million).

Table 1.2   **Average number of inpatient hospital stays and outpatient attendances per 100 persons in Great Britain in 1991**

Age	Inpatients		Outpatients	
	Male	Female	Male	Female
0–4	14	10	85	57
5–15	8	5	77	61
16–44	7	20	92	96
45–64	10	12	125	153
65–74	20	14	158	155
75 and over	32	22	183	173

Table 1.3   **Percentages of men and women who visited a dentist in 1991 (after OPCS 1992)**

	Men	Women
Go for regular checkups	42	58
Only go with problems	35	22

Clearly the total number of GP visits made by women will be inflated because of family planning, pregnancy, childbirth and children. Nevertheless, the gender differences apparent from these figures are thought to highlight the way women use GPs (i.e. as a point of referral) and that men go more hesitantly (OPCS 1992). Some have argued of course that rather than men going too infrequently, it is women who go too often. However, our concerns here are less about the frequency of visits, and more about the attitude that underpins this behaviour.

Hospital inpatient stays and outpatient attendances in 1991 show men in the majority in four of six age groupings (see Table 1.2), tending to suggest that men leave health matters unattended to longer than women.

Dental care statistics provide further evidence of this tendency (see Table 1.3). Few people like to go to the dentist, so regular checkups are a good indicator of a health mentality. While the 'regular checkup' percentages in Table 1.3 may be distorted by pregnancy, childbirth and children, this is unlikely to influence the 'only with problems' figures.

Living with a female partner appears to improve a man's health. Marriage (or living with a female partner) is thought to act as a protection from ill health. Other men, particularly separated and divorced men, have significantly higher mortality and morbidity rates. Widowed, divorced and separated men are also more likely to risk their health by, for example, smoking and drinking excessively. There are no comparable data for homosexual couples, so whether it is being in a relationship per se, or being in a relationship with a woman that protects men from ill health is difficult to determine (Gove 1979).

As mentioned above, many men have much more difficulty asking for help than women. Good, Dell & Mintz (1989) found that men felt they needed to be in control and self-sufficient, which often stopped them from asking for external help. In a survey of over 20 000 young people, Baldings asked: 'If you wanted to share health problems, to whom would you probably turn?' (Baldings 1993). He found that the answer 'no-one' came from:

- 12.8% of 12-year-old boys (compared with 6.9% of girls)
- 13.8% of 15-year-old boys (5.8% of girls).

When asked: 'When you have a problem, what do you do about it?', 18.8% of 12-year-old boys answered that they 'do nothing'. Briscoe (1989) suggests that:

> from an early age, girls become orientated towards the tendency to seek medical care for a wide variety of complaints, whereas boys learn to disregard pain and avoid doctors; hence an association is formed between being feminine and being more concerned with health.

To summarise, we can say that research has shown that the male gender role leads men to ignore their health needs. Men's attitudes and behaviours can be described as follows:

- Men perceive their bodies as machines.

- Men's health behaviours and beliefs are influenced by their perceptions of themselves as men.

- Men, on the whole, do not use health services in the same way as women, and tend to leave intervention until later.

- Living with a female partner improves a man's health.

- Many men don't see the need for help, or have more difficulty asking for it.

- Many men report that being employed conflicts with their health needs.

The consequences for practice

We have seen how men's attitudes and behaviours affect their health, and throw up specific needs. How can we use this knowledge to develop effective men's health initiatives? The following list provides some useful starting points to help us consider this question.

- *Addressing men's health requires an understanding of the barriers experienced by men and, importantly, by the professionals working with them.* It is all too easy for professionals to externalise issues such as men's use of primary health care services, and view them as being the men's problem only. Professionals often have stereotyped views, fixed assumptions (e.g. 'men cannot express emotions') that inhibit men's willingness to use services.

- *Primary healthcare (PHC) services have, on the whole, developed with the needs of women and children in mind.* Opening hours are a good indicator of the priorities of many PHC services. Daytime surgeries are the norm, and evening surgeries often operate without an appointment system, leading to longer waiting times.

- *We need to see men as responsible for their health, rather than women being the gatekeepers to family (including men's) health.* Until recently, if we wanted to target men, we targeted women (wives, partners or mothers), on the assumption that talking to the men directly would be less effective.

- *An understanding of masculinity will help us to target and deal with men much more effectively.* An increased understanding of masculinities, and of the fact that at any one time there may be a number of sometimes competing masculinities operating (Connell 1995), will help us think through targeting, the barriers for men and help our clinical practice.

■ *Having a positive approach to men (as patients) will help us work more effectively with men.* Given the choice, women will choose to see a woman doctor four times out of five. Men, however, are much more concerned about the doctor's regard towards them, and are less concerned about his or her gender.

■ *What do we know about the target group of men?* One of the major problems when targeting men is that we often know so little about them. This problem is increased because men do not necessarily use PHC services, so our opportunities to find out more are restricted.

■ *How can we find out more?* Where services have made a point of finding out more about their target grouping, their effectiveness has increased considerably. Women's health, and initiatives with gay men in relation to HIV/AIDS are good examples of this.

■ *Men's and women's healthcare initiatives are not in competition with one another.* Limited overall resources inevitably lead to priorities being identified, and men's and women's healthcare provision will be part of this process. However, too often men's and women's health are perceived as being in competition with one another. This attitude is unhelpful and unnecessary.

■ *Gender and sexism are different but overlapping concepts.* One of the problems in the field of men's and women's health is that the issue of gender has often either been seen as referring exclusively to women's health (Farrell 1994) or as being the same as sexism. In fact, the term gender is used when defining differences between men's and women's health, whereas sexism relates to the power imbalance between men and women.

■ *Men express their masculinity in diverse ways and this needs to be taken into account when working with men.* The appearance, with reasonable sales figures, of such magazines as *Men's Health* (and more lifestyle versions such as *GQ* and *Maxim*) indicates a growing interest in health on the part of some men (see Ch. 9). The readership of these magazines is young, on the whole from social class groups I and II, and has both aspirations and money. Many of these readers will use their health interest in ways which demonstrate and prove their masculinity, e.g. looking good, toned and more appealing to women and other men. For other men, this reflection of masculinity has little or no interest. Then there are those men whose aspirations and motivations may be completely different. They may be overweight, drink and smoke and know they are taking extensive risks, but they are not concerned with how such behaviour will affect them (though they may be concerned that their death or time off sick would affect their family).

■ *Men's lives are changing, and men are much more prepared to reflect on and discuss their health needs.* Unemployment, changing employment patterns, and the breaking-down of attitudes towards fixed gender roles (Lloyd 1997) have all contributed to men's increased willingness to address masculinity and its effects on their health. If health workers initiate discussion in this area, men tend, on the whole, to respond.

Men's health services

In Chapter 5, Fletcher offers a useful definition of a men's health service. It is one which:
1. addresses men's health issues
2. pays particular attention to targeting males, engaging males or treating males
3. incorporates an acknowledgement that existing services, whatever their merits, require a fresh approach to males' health in order to improve males' health status.

This definition encourages us to move away from one-dimensional strategies (such as men's health clinics) towards the more complex, multifaceted approach that the new public health agenda requires.

To illustrate the changes the new public health agenda may bring to men's health, we shall examine the issue of suicide.

Male suicide

Trends in suicide have dramatically increased for young men since the 1970s. Highlighted by the Chief Medical Officer

(Calman 1993), suicide has since received substantial interest and attention as a 'men's issue'. Charlton et al (1993) examined the incidence of suicide among men and concluded that the increase was:

> related to a complex set of social, economic, and other changes ... we suggest that the increasing number of men remaining single or becoming divorced may explain up to one-half of the increase in suicides observed between the early 1970s and late 80s. This age-group of men has also been affected by high unemployment rates, exposure to armed combat, increasing risk of imprisonment, an increase in misuse of alcohol and other drugs, and the HIV virus. There is little evidence of a rise in the prevalence of mental illness.

Charlton and colleagues were unable to find a correlation between changes in unemployment and suicide rates, although Pritchard (1992) did. In a study of men in Oxford, Hawton et al (1989) suggested that while unemployment was rarely a direct cause of attempted suicide, there may be indirect association via factors such as psychological vulnerability, or the problems brought on by unemployment (such as poverty). A Liverpool study of young men and suicide (Stanistreet 1996) hypothesised that a:

> lack of integration into society results in low social status, inadequate practical and social support and a poor quality of social environment, leading to increased life stressors, increased hopelessness and dissatisfaction with life, increased anger and a tendency towards self-destructive behaviour.

The literature reviewed here provides us with enough indicators of cause to point to a clear target group and a number of quite specific areas for action. This in itself is unusual with health research and practice. If we were to review coronary heart disease in the same way, for instance, we would have more difficulties finding clear areas for action, and studies that addressed gender and successful interventions. While all of these are important components within a public health framework, it has been argued that the number of suicide deaths is not high enough to warrant attention as a specific target, and that improved mental health would be a better target to aim for. It may be the case that numbers affected will become the overall criterion for targeting. Nevertheless, let us continue with our current example. Addressing men's suicide effectively may involve the following wider issues:

- increasing the number of catalytic converters on cars
- accelerating the introduction of paracetamol blister packs
- increasing the number and quality of jobs available
- reducing crime and the fear of crime
- developing men's networks to replace those lost in the workplace
- developing strategies to enable men to ask for help
- developing 'safety net' services for men (such as crisis lines, post-redundancy and unemployment mental health programmes in and outside of the workplace)
- increasing funding for the Samaritans, and other suicide prevention agencies such as the National Farmers Union phoneline.

And within health services, the following are possible areas of action:

- developing quality mental health services that incorporate an awareness of men and suicide
- developing drug addiction programmes further, including an awareness of men and suicide
- raising awareness of men and suicide with HIV and AIDS practitioners
- developing prison mental health services
- developing school-based programmes for boys in 'feeling, recognition and expression', 'self-esteem' and 'suicide prevention'
- developing the abilities of primary healthcare and other professionals to identify those young men who are at risk.

Conclusion

In this chapter we have presented:

- statistical data
- a brief review of literature
- a layered review of the changing context
- some starting points
- a definition and an illustration of what a men's health service may look like.

Of course, the broadening context in which we think about men's health also highlights the lack of research and data on men, their health and effective strategies and practice. If we are to consider aspects outside of the individual, we must develop an adequate research and data base. We must also develop adequate evaluation methods and highlight good examples of practice. The reason suicide was selected to illustrate a public health strategy was that other targets such as CHD lack a gender focus in the research, although the epidemiological evidence does exist. This provides a very shaky base for strategy development, especially with such a broad canvas. However, services and intervention have to start somewhere and in this book we offer a number of initiatives that we would define as being well within the confines of men's health.

References

Ashton J, Seymour H 1988 The new public health. Open University Press, Milton Keynes

Baldings J 1993 Young people in 1992. Schools Health Education Unit, University of Exeter

Bem S 1987 The measurement of psychological androgyny. Journal of Consulting and Clinical Psychology 42:155–162

Blaxter M 1990 Health and lifestyles. Routledge, London

Bray R et al 1997 Can boys do better? Secondary Heads Association, Leicester

Brenner M 1979 Mortality and the national economy. Lancet 2:568–569

Briscoe, M E 1989 Sex differences in mental health. Update, 1st November: 834–839

Burgess A, Ruxton S 1996 Men and their children. IPPR, London

Burghes L, Clarke L, Cronin N 1997 Fathers and fatherhood in Britain. Family Policy Studies Centre, London

Calman K 1993 On the state of the public health – 1992. HMSO, London

Charlton J, Kelly S, Dunnell K, Evans B, Jenkins R, Wallis R 1993 Suicide deaths in England and Wales: trends in factors associated with suicide deaths. Population Trends 71(Spring):34–43

Clarke M, Hunter D J, Wistow G 1997 For debate: Local government and the National Health Service: the new agenda. Journal of Public Health Medicine 19(1):3–5

Cohen P 1998a View from the bridge. Healthlines December 97–January 98:17–19

Cohen P 1998b Health matters for local authorities. Healthlines February:13–15

Connell R W 1995 Masculinities. Polity Press, Cambridge

Davis F, Walsh W B 1988 Antecedents and consequences of gender role conflict: an empirical test of sex role strain analysis. Paper presented at the 96th Annual Convention of the APA, Atlanta, GA

Dench G 1996 The place of men in changing family cultures. Institute of Community Studies, London

Department of Education 1993 HMSO, London

Department of Employment 1997 Labour force survey. HMSO, London

Department of Health 1998a Government Actuary's. HMSO, London

Department of Health 1998b Our healthier nation: a contract for health. HMSO, London

Derlega V J, Winstead B A, Jones W H 1991 Personality: contemporary theory and research. Nelson-Hall, Chicago

Drever F, Whitehead M (eds) 1997 Health inequalities. Office for national statistics, HMSO, London

Edley N, Wetherell M 1995 Men in perspective. Prentice Hall, London

Farad A 1994 Equal rights for men. Nursing Times 90:26–29

Farrell, W 1994 The myth of male power. The 4th Estate, London

Fitzgerald L F, Cherpas C C 1985 On the reciprocal relationship between gender and occupation: rethinking the assumptions concerning masculine career development. Journal of Vocational Behaviour 27:109–122

Gabby J 1998 Our healthier nation. British Medical Journal 316:487–488

Giddens A 1993 Sociology. Polity Press, Cambridge

Gilmore D D 1990 Manhood in the making: cultural concepts of masculinity. Yale University Press, Newhaven

Good G E, Dell D M, Mintz L B 1989 Male role and gender role conflict: relations to help seeking in men. Journal of Counselling and Psychotherapy 36(3):295–300

Gove W 1979 Sex, marital status and mortality. American Journal of Sociology 45–67

Government Statistical Service 1990 Criminal statistics England and Wales. HMSO, London

Hanson J 1984 Sex education for young children. Journal of Marriage and the Family 42

Haviland M G, Shaw D G, Cummings M A, MacMurrey J P 1988 The relationship between alexithymia and depressive symptoms in a sample of newly alcoholic inpatients. Psychotherapy and Psychosomatics 50:81–87

Hawton K et al 1989 Alcoholism, alcohol and attempted suicide. Alcohol and Alcoholism 24(1):3–9

HMSO 1991 Key area handbook on accidents. HMSO, London

HMSO 1993 Annual abstract of statistics. HMSO, London

Home Office 1994a Criminal statistics for England and Wales. HMSO, London

Home Office 1994b Statistical bulletin 10/94. HMSO, London

Home Office 1997 Criminal statistics. HMSO, London

Kilmartin C T 1994 The masculine self. Macmillan, New York

Kimmel M S 1994 Masculinity as homophobia: fear, shame and silence in the construction of gender identity. In: Brod H, Kaufman M (eds) Theorizing masculinities. Sage, Los Angeles

Klein A 1995 Life's too short to die small. In: Sabo D, Gordon D F (eds) Men's health and illness. Sage, London

Lau et al 1986 Health as a value; methodological and theoretical considerations. Health Psychology 5:25–43

Lewis T 1988 Unemployment and men's health. Nursing 3(26)

Lloyd T J 1996 A review of men's health. RCN, London

Lloyd T J 1997 Let's get changed lads. Working With Men, London

Long V O 1989 Relation of masculinity to self-esteem and self-acceptance in male professionals, college students, and scientists. Journal of Counselling Psychology 36:84–87

Macintyre S 1990 Gender differences in the perceptions of common cold symptom. Social Science Medicine 36(1):15–20

Manuk S B, Polefrone J M 1987 Psychophysiologic reactivity in women. In: Eaker E D et al (eds) Coronary heart disease in women. Haymarket Doyma, New York

O'Dowd T, Jewell D 1998 Men's health. Oxford University Press, Oxford

O'Neil J M 1990 Assessing men's gender role conflict. In: Moore D, Leafgren F (eds) Men and Conflict. American Association of Counselling and Development, Alexandria, VA

OPCS 1992 General household survey. HMSO, London

OPCS 1994 General household survey. HMSO, London

Orr J 1987 Women's health in the community. John Wiley, Chichester

Ounsted M 1972 Gender and intrauterine growth with a note on the sex proband as a research tool. In: Ounsted C & Taylor D C (eds) Gender differences: their ontogeny and significance. Churchill Livingstone, Edinburgh

Pleck J 1981 The myth of masculinity. MIT Press, Cambridge, MA

Pritchard C 1992 Is there a link between suicide in young men and unemployment, a comparison of the UK with other European Community Countries. British Journal of Psychiatry 160:750–756

Ramsey E R, Ramwell P 1984 The relationship of the sex hormone/prostaglandin interaction to female and male longevity. In: Gold E B (ed) The changing risk of disease in women: an epidemiologic approach. Lexington, MA

Reddy D M, Fleming R, Adesso V J 1992 Gender and health. International Review of Health Psychology 1:1–32

Robertson S 1995 Men's health promotion in the UK: a hidden problem. British Journal of Nursing 4(7)

Saltonstall R 1993 Healthy bodies, social bodies: men's and women's concepts and practices of health in everyday life. Social Science Medicine 36(1):7–14

Skelton R 1988 Man's role in society and its effect on health. Nursing 3(26)

Stanistreet D 1996 Injury and poisoning mortality among young men. Working With Men 3:16–18

Templer D I, Griffin P R, Hintze J 1993 Gender life expectancy and alcohol: an international perspective. International Journal of Addictions 28:1613–1620

The Sunday Times 1998 Blair tackles men behaving badly. 3 May

The Sunday Times, 19 June 1994

Verbrugge L M 1985 Gender and health: an update of hypotheses and evidence. Journal of Health and Social Behaviour 26:156–182

Waldron I 1988 Gender and health-related behaviour. In: Gochman D S (ed) Health behaviour: emerging research perspectives. Plenum Press, New York

Warden J 1998 Britain's new health policy recognises poverty as major cause of illness. British Medical Journal 316:495

Watson J M 1993 Male body image and health beliefs: a qualitative study and implications for health promotion practice. Health Education Journal 52(4)

Weitzman L 1972 Sexual socialization in picture books for preschool children. American Journal of Sociology 77

Wingard D L 1984 The sex differential in morbidity, mortality and lifestyle. Annual Review Public Health 5:433–458

Wingard D L 1984 The sex differential in morbidity, mortality and lifestyle. Annual Review of Public Health 5:433–458

2

Inequalities in men's health

Siân Griffiths

This chapter covers:

- inequalities
- mortality differences between men and women
- suicide
- mortality differences between men
- morbidity differences between men and women.

Introduction

Inequalities in health are the result of a variety of factors – social, economic environmental, individual. Comparative statistics on the health of men and women show that men in the UK:

- die on average 6 years younger than women
- are three-and-a-half times more likely to die from coronary heart disease under 65
- have a suicide rate at least double that of women
- are more likely to smoke, drink and be overweight
- are more likely to contract HIV/AIDS.

These statistics reflect higher levels of risk-taking, which are also shown in men's use of healthcare and their health behaviours. As has been shown in Chapter 1, men are less likely to turn up for their health checks than women, and are more likely to have become severely ill by the time they get to their doctor. They are less likely to take active steps to improve their health. But the differentials are not just between men and women but between different groups of men – based on differences in

income, occupation and ethnic group. This chapter will explore
some of these differences for men in the UK.

Inequalities

Inequalities in health are not a new phenomenon. The links
between wealth and health were well recognised across history.
As early as the 16th century there were differential death rates
between babies born in poor parts of London, where 30 out of
every 100 could expect to survive to 15, compared to 69 out of
every 100 amongst ducal families. The sanitary reformers of the
19th century recognised the importance of clean air, water and
hygiene in addressing the health of the poor.

However, it has not always been politically acceptable to
highlight the impact of social and environmental factors on
health. Successive Conservative Governments of the 1980s and
1990s fought shy of recognising the impact of social factors –
and hence policy – on health: first in the suppression of the Black
report (Black et al 1980) and then again using the word 'variations' rather than 'inequalities' in the Department of Health
report of 1995 (Department of Health 1995). The Chief Medical
Officer of England had, however, been explicit in his annual
report about the impact of poverty on ill health (Calman 1995).

With the change of Government in 1997 the importance of
redressing inequalities in health by tackling the broader determinants such as housing and employment became recognised in
a variety of policy initiatives – not least the establishment of the
Social Exclusion Unit in Downing Street and by the launch of
Green Papers. For example *Our healthier nation* (Department
of Health 1998) shifts the emphasis away from the focus on
individual lifestyle characteristics towards the interaction of
individuals and their socioeconomic environment. This
acknowledges that although individual determinants such as
genetic and behavioural characteristics are important, the
environment in which people live has a key influence on their
health. Thus it is not only what one eats that is important, but
how food is distributed to communities. For example, eating
white bread may be the only option if it's all the shops near you
sell or all that you can afford. The solution is not just to exhort
you to eat brown bread because it's better for you, but to make
sure it is available at reasonable prices.

Addressing inequalities in health by 'joining up' the policies from different sectors of society is a fundamental task in improving health. Against this background it is interesting to ask how well men fare, and which men fare best.

Mortality differences between men and women

In his annual report for 1992, the Chief Medical Officer of England described the different health profiles for men and women, highlighting that although more boys were born – 106 male for every 100 female births – males had consistently higher mortality (Calman 1993). Fetal mortality was higher amongst males, and the 20% higher pattern of infant mortality was reflected in all ages thereafter. In 1991 an 18-year-old man had an 80% chance of surviving to his 65th birthday; an 18-year-old woman's chances were 88%. In subsequent reports the improving health of men has been revealed. By 1995, average male life expectancy had risen to 74.3 years, with a projected rise to 75.5 years by 2001–2002 (Calman 1997).

Comparing mortality rates for men and women in the same report we see that more young men died from causes such as accidents, suicide and AIDS. There was also a peak at around 65 years of age, due to higher male death rates from coronary heart disease and lung cancer. 70% of all male deaths in 1992 were as a result of circulatory diseases and cancers. Causes of male deaths vary, as would be expected, with age. Road accident related deaths in 1992 were highest amongst men of 15–34, accounting for one-fifth of the deaths in this age group. Looking in more detail at causes of death for men aged 20–64, one-third were from neoplasms (cancers), almost two-fifths from diseases of the circulatory system and around one-eighth from external causes of injury and poisoning.

Some of the major causes of male mortality are targeted in *Our healthier nation* (Department of Health 1998). These include:

- smoking
- coronary heart disease
- road traffic accidents
- suicide.

Smoking

The most common killers are heart disease and lung cancer. Both are related to smoking tobacco, and men have traditionally smoked more than women. However, trends are changing. In 1972 the death rate from lung cancer was five times higher for men than for women – but by 1992 it was only twice as high. This is a clear demonstration of the impact of changing lifestyles on health. The General Household Survey of 1994 found that 28% of men and 26% of women smoked (Hawton 1992). In 1974, the figures were 51% of men and 41% of women. Although more men than women smoke, more men will have tried and succeeded in giving up. Until Richard Doll's work examining smoking in doctors, which linked tobacco with lung cancer, male doctors had high rates of smoking. Now it is rare to find male doctors who smoke. Worryingly, the numbers of young women smokers is rising.

Coronary heart disease

Coronary heart disease is a major killer, killing more men than women. It is closely related to individual lifestyle factors such as smoking, and to direct, social and environmental influences. Reducing deaths in the under-65s is a key Government target.

Road traffic accidents

One of the areas of risk-taking that kills disproportionately more young men is road traffic accidents. In 1992, three-quarters of deaths from accidental injuries were men between the ages of 15 and 64. 46% of accidental deaths in men were due to motor vehicle accidents, and young men were more likely than young women to have accidents when driving. Risk-taking behaviour, combined with lack of experience, alcohol intake and, to a lesser extent, drug use, are significant causes of accidents in this group.

Suicide

Suicide is associated not only with previously diagnosed mental illness but also with a variety of social factors. Hawton (1992) emphasises that we need to consider the concept 'suicide' as a spectrum, which ranges from vague thoughts about suicide through more serious thoughts, a suicidal act either with little or no suicidal intent or considerable intent, to completed suicide.

For every one teenage suicide there are 100 attempts. It has been suggested that at some time 10–20% of teenagers entertain quite serious suicidal ideas. This is particularly worrying since between 1980 and 1990 the suicide rate in 15–64-year-old males increased by 85%, most markedly amongst 20–24-year-olds. Hawton suggests that contributory factors include:

- rising rates of unemployment
- increasing alcohol and drug abuse
- increasing rates of family breakdown
- increasing availability of dangerous methods
- HIV/AIDS.

Mortality differences between men

Mortality rates do not only vary between men and women. As one would suspect, men themselves do not form a homogeneous group. Research has shown that in England and Wales, men in social class V have almost three times the mortality, and those in classes IIIM and IV nearly twice the mortality of men in class I (Drever & Whitehead 1997). Young men between 20 and 24 from class V experience the same mortality rates as class I men 20 years older. The class differentials for stroke, lung cancer, accidents and suicides are even greater – and the differentials between classes I and V have widened since the 1970s, despite an overall downward trend. In other words, affluent men are more healthy than their less well-off counterparts, and are getting healthier at a faster rate.

Looking at the figures in more detail, we see that:

- Mortality from heart disease and stroke is twice that of England and Wales as a whole, and three times that of men in class I (part of this difference is associated with higher smoking rates in class V).

- Mortality from accidents and suicides is four times greater in social class V than in class I reflected particularly in motor vehicle accidents, which are three times more common in men in class V.

- Men who are unemployed are over twice as likely as employed men to commit suicide, and men who are single, widowed or divorced are three times as likely. (Further analysis of unemployment and mortality suggests that there is an independent effect of unemployment on mortality, not explained by other factors such as marital status).

- Men with AIDS, men in prison and abusers of drugs and alcohol are also more likely to commit suicide.

Further analysis of this report shows that there are different rates of male mortality amongst migrant groups. This is partly due to the higher proportions of manual workers, but this is not the whole story. There are also different patterns of mortality amongst the different ethnic groups. For example, Irish and Scottish men show higher mortality from accidents, injuries and suicide, whereas men born in East Africa and the Indian subcontinent show higher mortality from ischaemic heart disease. The association between social class and migrant status is not clear cut. Mortality for all men in a manual class is 30% higher than the general rate for all men, but the figure for all men born on the Indian subcontinent is twice the national rate. Men born in the Caribbean experience lower mortality from ischaemic heart disease. In their analysis of the differences in mortality amongst migrants Harding & Maxwell (1997) concluded that social class is not an adequate explanation for the excess mortality in men from minority ethnic groups. They refer to studies in the US which have begun to explore the complex mechanisms, such as failed job improvement and work-related stress, through which social disadvantage may contribute to differences in survival between blacks and whites.

The growing differentials in male mortality are not well understood, but it is likely that factors such as increased social stress from economic insecurity, lack of secure employment and changing social expectations impact negatively on less affluent men. There seems little way out of the poverty trap for many, and this can lead to risk-taking behaviours which can be seen as both a means of expression and a symptom of alienation.

Morbidity differences between men and women

It is not only death rates that reflect differences between the health of men and women and between different groups of men. Morbidity and health behaviours, although difficult to measure, also show different patterns.

Available data show that for most illnesses men are less likely than women to consult their general practitioners, yet their hospital admission rates for diseases such as coronary heart disease and stroke are higher. Men are more likely to wait until their symptoms are more severe before seeking help, and they are less likely to attend health checks or dental checks. Studies of long-term sickness show that there are no significant differences in the proportions of men and women who report chronic or long-standing illness. However, men in lower socio-economic groups are more likely to define their health as fair or poor than either women in comparable groups or men in higher socioeconomic groups.

Some common diseases show different patterns. For example, statistics show that men are less likely to suffer from depression or anxiety than women, but are as likely to be diagnosed schizophrenic. The diagnosis is more likely to be made at a younger age in men – peaking at between 15 and 24. Particular groups of men are more likely to be severely mentally ill. This includes the homeless. More than ten times as many men as women live in hostels for the homeless, and 30–50% of them suffer from severe mental illness. Young African-Caribbean men are more likely to suffer from severe mental illness and to be admitted to secure wards. Commenting on these and other statistics, Chan (1995) suggests that improvement in the health of men from ethnic minorities will depend on the reduction of stress generated by unemployment, poor housing and other forms of racism, as reflected in the suicide statistics particularly for young men.

Another disease which affects men more than women in the UK is HIV/AIDS. The majority of men in the UK who become infected are men who have had sex with men. However, statistics show that the proportion of cases of HIV/AIDS infection acquired from sex between men has been falling (to 64% in 1997) whereas infection from sex between women and men had risen to 30%.

Substance abuse is more common in men than in women. Nearly 90% of boys in the UK have drunk alcohol by the time they are 13. 25% of 13–17 year-olds get into arguments and fights after drinking alcohol and 1000 children under 15 are admitted to hospital each year with acute alcohol poisoning (Macfarlane 1996). Alcohol is a contributory cause of road traffic accidents. Alcohol abuse correlates strongly with accidents and with crime. About one-fifth of convicted prisoners, the vast majority of them male, have an alcohol or drug-related problem. Alcohol is implicated as a factor in 60% of murders, 75% of stabbings, 70% of beatings, 40% of domestic violence incidents and 20% of child abuse – most of these offences being committed by men. Prisoners are four times as likely as their peer group to describe themselves as drinking 'quite a lot' or as drinking 'heavily'. A study by Gunn (1992) found that 8.6% of sentenced prisoners had a primary diagnosis of alcohol dependence or abuse, and Maden et al (1996) found that 15.4% of remand prisoners were alcohol-dependent.

Drug misuse is also associated with crime, and three-quarters of opioid addicts notified to the Home Office are men. 75% of registered drug misusers have a criminal record, usually related to drug use. In 1988 half the drug offenders in the UK were aged between 21 and 29, and 88% of them were men.

Conclusion

Changing men's health behaviours poses a challenge. Statistics show that the men who are hearing health messages are unlikely to be those at greatest risk – who, even if they hear, may well not be motivated to act. To address the growing gap in health inequalities, more needs to be done about the fundamental causes of ill health, which lie in the social environment.

The links between poverty and ill health are clear. The links between drugs, crime, violence, imprisonment, unemployment and men's ill health highlight the need to educate young men, rather than to concentrate exclusively on promoting lifestyle changes for the motivated. Recognition that there is a shift away from manual tasks towards more technological and computerised means of production has led to national initiatives to re-skill men who might previously have earned their living from manual labour. This represents a step in the right direction, as the root cause of many of the inequalities in men's health is the lack of employment and resources to live in a way which would result in better health.

Re-addressing the inequalities in men's health requires composite effort from those constructing the social and economic environment, as well as efforts by individuals to adopt healthy lifestyles. Both the risks men take in their lifestyles, and the risky social environment in which they live need to be addressed if their health is to be improved.

References

Black D, Morris N, Smith C, Townsend P 1980 Inequalities in health: a report of a Research Working Group. DHSS London

Calman K 1993 On the state of the public health – 1992. HMSO, London, pp 79–107

Calman K 1995 On the state of the public health – 1994. HMSO, London

Calman K 1997 On the state of the public health – 1996. HMSO, London

Chan M 1995 Ethnicity and men's health. Report of conference: Men's Health Matters. The Medicine Group

Department of Health 1995 Variations in health. HMSO, London

Department of Health 1998 Our healthier nation. HMSO, London

Dever F, Whitehead M (eds) 1997 Health inequalities. HMSO, London

Gunn J 1992 Personality disorders and forensic psychiatry. Criminal Behaviour and Mental Health 2:202–211

Harding S, Maxwell R 1997 Differences in mortality of migrants. In: Dever F, Whitehead M (eds) Health inequalities. HMSO, London, pp 27–29

Hawton K 1992 By their own hand. British Medical Journal 304:1000

Macfarlane A 1996 The user: drug use by young people. OUP, Oxford, pp 27–29

Maden A, Taylor C, Brooke D, Gunn J 1996 Mental disorders in remand prisoners. Institute of Psychiatry, London

3

Commissioning and men: the case of STDs

Lindsay Neil

This chapter covers:

- commissioning
- sexually transmitted diseases
- the case of gonorrhoea among gay men
- the present: gonorrhoea today
- the future: a hypothetical case study.

Introduction

The principle of separating the 'thinkers' from the 'doers' in the NHS (what has been called the purchaser–provider split) is now well established and referred to as 'commissioning'.

Commissioning decisions heavily influence the practice of health promotion. Part 2 of this book presents many examples of effective ways of working directly with men. This chapter looks higher up the chain, at how commissioning decisions are made.

Commissioning strategies are considerably less well developed than practice. Good decision-making at this level is essential. Like any design, if the foundations are not strong, the purpose will be limited at best, and in the worst cases, may even be counterproductive.

This chapter examines commissioning in the context of men and sexually transmitted diseases (STDs). The principles discussed here are applicable to all men's health issues.

Commissioning

Commissioning decisions themselves are heavily dependent on the availability of good information. This is of course the case for all commissioning, but we find particular difficulties in the collection and use of data related to STDs. We will look here at the information which is available and which should be kick-starting the commissioning process, and consider why it is usually absent. Much of what we have to say here is as relevant to women as it is to men. However, there are a number of factors which make it important to consider men separately:

- Social constructs strongly affect male sexual behaviour and are the foundation of this book.

- In general, men remain the more powerful partner in heterosexual relationships, particularly with regard to sexual behaviour.

- A significant proportion of STDs among women come from their regular (and in many cases they believe their monogamous) partner.

- Reducing STDs among gay men has had some success.

The significance of men's socialisation needs to be sufficiently understood by those responsible for commissioning. However, it would be unrealistic to expect any commissioner to have particular expertise – or even particular interest – beyond being able to identify when men need to be specifically targeted. Other chapters of this book explore the complexity of male socialisation and readers are urged to make use of those in pursuing the commissioning principles which are drawn out of the case studies presented here.

Taking gonorrhoea as an example, we have three devices for demonstrating the potential gains from commissioning. These are:

1. a past (successful) case study
2. the present situation
3. the future.

We explore the reasons for the present situation, and identify the barriers that are currently operating against repeating the strategy of the case study. Our guiding principles throughout are the need to be honest about what we know and modest about what we can achieve.

In order to take a strategic view, we are going to focus on disease rather than on (sexual) health, and we draw a distinction here between health promotion and disease prevention, and assume it is possible to reduce STDs. In the NHS, this requires the development of outcomes to measure the impact of investment in prevention. It has to be admitted that this will be a largely theoretical discussion, simply because establishing outcomes is particularly fraught with problems. These arise from a combination of:

- the collection and use of data
- findings from behavioural research
- medical treatment
- anxiety about stigmatising
- denials about sexual behaviour
- moral judgements,
- a widespread reluctance in general to be honest about what we do during our sexual careers.

We are not deterred by the 'challenges' posed here and neither are we apologetic about a largely theoretical discussion. We find an increasing willingness to address just these challenges, and we are happy to make our contribution.

Because of the social and cultural complexities of sexual behaviour, we have to call on a very broad range of approaches if we are to have any significant impact on the adverse consequences. This means that professionals have to act with the support and consensus of a larger variety of vested interests than, say, those working on reducing heart disease. Community commitment to prevention is desirable in all cases; in this one, it is crucial because the scope of the NHS cannot and should not extend into the personal lives of individuals and communities, and can never influence peer norms in the way that communities do.

Before we move into those specific areas, and mindful that readers will have very different professional experiences of STDs – and probably also about commissioning – we begin with some background information and comment.

Sexually transmitted diseases

Men get a bad press when it comes to STDs. The nature of the bad press ranges from allegations that they 'just don't care', through the notion that STDs are an inevitable bit of bad luck, to the more extreme view that having an STD is in fact proof of manhood. More invidiously, there are widely held assumptions about 'what sort of person' gets an STD, and gay men and black men are often presumed to make up most of the clients of any genitourinary (GU) clinic.

As with all stereotyping, there is some truth in each of those allegations. However, while the picture we get from these stereotypes may have echoes of truth, they also contain inaccuracies, and certainly take us nowhere in terms of understanding the socialisation of STDs. Without a clear and accurate picture it is impossible to identify, act on and demonstrate change. In this chapter we identify the type and sources of information available to us and consider some of the key barriers to the collection and application of this information. Further, we focus on prevention and not on treatment, although these two cannot easily be separated.

Commissioning offers the only opportunity to determine outcome measures and then to provide the resources for meeting them. However, in order to make best use of these, we have to be clear about a number of factors:

- we will never eliminate them
- we don't need to be 'promiscuous' to be caught by one (we are not offering a working definition of that widely used term)
- we are remarkably ignorant about STDs.

In the early 1990s, the Health Education Authority (HEA) ran a small survey to check levels of knowledge about STDs. From a list of 10, a surprising number of people had heard about the one called 'gonaditis'. What was particularly interesting about this, is that the disease was an invention of the (male) researcher. Somehow, being worried about your gonads seems to be a sensible thing.

There is an interesting imbalance between knowledge and experience. Our awareness of and knowledge about HIV is very high, and yet for the vast majority of the UK population, experience of it is likely to be nil. By contrast, other STDs are far more common – but the level of awareness and knowledge about them is very low.

We the population, then, know a lot less than we should about STDs, other than HIV. We need to be well-informed so that we can:

- better understand the risks we take
- recognise symptoms that need treatment and get it quickly
- appreciate the risks we pose to others if we have an STD
- be really helpful to any friends or family that either put themselves at risk or actually get caught
- generally have a more well-informed view of what these things are all about, and discard any prejudices and misunderstandings we have.

We dare to suggest that these points apply as much to professionals working 'in the field' as they do to the 'general population'.

It is also instructive, although not within our remit here, to know something of the historical and contemporary global patterns of STDs. Briefly, these include the claim that during the First World War, more hospital beds were occupied by men with 'venereal diseases' than men with war injuries. In more modern times, wherever there is social conflict, there is a significant increase in STDs, and these days that includes HIV. Migrant labour has been a major factor in the spread of HIV in Southern Africa and in India. It remains the case that many heterosexual relationships are unequal when it comes to sex, and that in some parts of the world a woman's greatest risk of STDs, including HIV, comes from her husband's sexual behaviour. Some of the poorest countries of the world have far higher rates of STDs than the UK, not because of marked differences in sexual behaviour, but because of marked differences in medical treatment.

Any singular view of STDs will distort the significance of the diseases themselves, and therefore our ability to minimise the damage they do. We have to see them for what they are: a longstanding, global, social, medical and public health problem.

We know we will never eliminate STDs. We know that over time, STDs can both increase and decrease according to our ability to treat them effectively. We know that we will never stop the sexual behaviour that keeps STDs moving among us. Remember: honesty and modesty!

At this point, we go on to look at the first of the three devices mentioned on page 48, which will serve to illustrate the potential gains to be derived from commissioning.

The case of gonorrhoea among gay men

This is a success story. Although it predates 'commissioning', it is based on honesty and modesty, and makes the best use of the information available at the time. Before examining the issues though, it is important to clarify a few points concerning terminology. There is considerable debate about what words are appropriate to denote men who have sex with men. In the context of sexuality, 'gay' is a social construct and not a description of sexual behaviour. It therefore excludes men having sex with men who would not identify themselves as gay, but as heterosexual, or possibly bisexual. There is research which suggests that there are men who have sex with men and who do not ascribe any sexuality to themselves. However, for the purposes of illustrating our point here, we are using the term 'gay men' expressly because of its social construct.

So, to return to our case study. Symptoms of gonorrhoea show relatively soon after infection and treatment is fairly straightforward. All cases in England are compulsorily reported directly to the Centre for Communicable Disease Surveillance (CCDC); cases in Scotland are reported to the Scottish CCDC. The forms used by GU clinics for collecting these data (called KC60 forms) ask if the infection is believed to have been 'homosexually acquired'. Whilst it is unlikely that this section is always filled in correctly, the numbers of reported 'homosexually acquired' gonorrhoea cases in the 1980s were high, and were the cause of a significant burden of ill health among gay men. This was the first of the available facts.

The second fact was identified through research which showed that the presence of gonorrhoea increased the effectiveness of HIV transmission. It followed therefore that treatment of gonorrhoea would reduce to some extent a man's risk of being infected with HIV.

The third fact was that it was shown that gonorrhoea was transmitted in the same ways as HIV, but became visible a great deal sooner.

In *The health of the nation* (Department of Health 1992) gonorrhoea was identified as a marker for HIV, and targets were set for the reduction of gonorrhea. Making best use of all the available data, and responding to very real anxieties about HIV within the communities, campaigns were run to alert gay men to the significance of the disease. A large helping of courage was added to the strict facts, and these campaigns were the first to be developed directly with the involvement of gay men themselves, making use of dedicated media, social venues and community networks. There were criticisms, at the time and since, that the involvement was not as strong as it could or should be. Certainly, the UK model falls some way short of the gay community led pro-grammes now common in Australia, the only country yet to show a reduction in HIV among gay men. Nevertheless, in the UK, this and subsequent campaigns depended on the collaboration of the target group. In the late 1980s and early 1990s, gonorrhoea cases among gay men declined dramatically.

The reduction of STDs in general is now extensively used to underpin HIV prevention programmes worldwide. Rigorous research in a number of countries (notably Uganda) confirms that, as a strategy, STD reduction significantly and rapidly reduces the number of HIV infections.

The principles for commissioning which we draw from this very brief description of our case study are:

- data and research have to be made public
- information has to be widely disseminated and discussed within the communities affected
- the sexual behaviour which leads to STDs has to be made explicit (thankfully it is some time since we have seen coy terms used about transmission through 'bodily fluids'!)
- campaigns and programmes must be developed with (and we mean with, not for) the communities affected.

To a large extent, these principles now apply to the vast majority of HIV and other STD prevention work with gay men. There does however, remain concern about how to apply those principles to men who are having sex with men and who do not see themselves as gay.

The present: gonorrhoea today

Despite the successful reduction of gonorrhoea in the incidence among gay men in the UK and the 1992 *Health of the nation* target, we are still left with a large (and in some regions increasing) caseload of the disease. The vast majority of these infections are no longer identified as 'homosexually acquired'. There appears to be an intense reluctance on the part of health authorities to release the data which would shed light on just what types of people are currently being infected, and how.

In addition to the KC60 forms mentioned above, GU clinics also collect data about their patients such as:

- age
- sex
- ethnic group (by self-classification)
- postcode
- validated district of residence
- diagnosis group (as the KC60 forms)
- whether attendance is a 'new' attendance.

Furthermore, all GU clinics have health advisers who are given a considerable number of personal details by their clients. In many if not most cases, the health adviser will gain some information about the circumstances in which the infection probably happened.

However, it is extraordinarily difficult for researchers outside the GU departments as well as service providers to get access to any of this information. As a result, our picture remains very fuzzy, and it is virtually impossible to develop outcome measures against which to judge the effectiveness of any investment.

To summarise then, the current gonorrhoea situation is at best static and in some places increasing. We know that gay men feature very much less in this profile than they used to. We are left with the question then, who else is in there?

The four principles of effective commissioning that we learnt from the gay men's case study above are markedly absent from commissioning for any other population group. A number of reasons for this are put forward, which need to be acknowledged. However, it is our view that none of them stand up when compared with the willingness to be open and candid about STDs and gay men. Let us be frank about some of these reasons.

■ *It is known that in some areas, African-Caribbean men are hugely over-represented in the gonorrhoea figures (in one clinic serving a community where African-Caribbean people make up 4% of the population, they represent nearly 50% of the gonorrhoea cases).* It is far more contentious to write this than it has ever been to claim that lots of gay men have had gonorrhoea. And yet we have never been able to prove that gay men are over-represented in the figures, because there is no 'Sexuality Census' equivalent to the 1991 Population Census. We have no way of knowing, or at least no way of agreeing, what percentage of us are hetero- or homosexual.

■ *Secrecy about the data is often disguised as confidentiality.* In some clinics the actual number of STD cases is small, and there is concern that providing too much profile detail will compromise confidentiality. Similarly, in areas with very small numbers of minority communities, identifying them in local data could compromise confidentiality. However, in the majority of areas, it is perfectly possible to produce anonymised data for commissioning purposes.

■ *Minority communities often deny the existence amongst their numbers of those behaviours, particularly sexual, which they believe reflect badly on their members or contradict their religious, cultural or philosophical beliefs.* Common examples of this would include sex before or outside marriage (paid for or free), homosexuality or any anal sex, and injecting drug use. However, all the research, historical texts, cultural artefacts and anecdotal evidence available to us clearly point to these behaviours being worldwide.

■ *Men tend to have an ambivalence about notions of fidelity, monogamy and numbers of sexual partners.* STD prevention can only operate in that gap between the public and the private which we know is so crucial to the behaviour of men. Elsewhere, the implications of this are discussed for the many behaviours which create problems for men, and therefore for us all.

The future: a hypothetical case study

This is the easy bit .... If, as we hope, the case for modesty and honesty has been made, it only remains for local commissioners and communities to exchange what they know and to agree on the need to reduce gonorrhoea. The gap between the present situation and the agreed outcomes is where prevention will happen. The effectiveness of this prevention will rely heavily on new partnerships between those who have the responsibility for the proper investment of public money, and the men who are directly affected by STDs, who are the only ones who can affect the behaviour change necessary. And this is also where the differences between the public claims and the private beliefs of men operate so powerfully.

If all this sounds rather bold, we conclude with a couple of reassurances, based on experience. Firstly, remember that it has been possible to be honest, modest and effective in reducing gonorrhoea among gay men. Secondly, our experience is that communities are more angry about a major health problem being ignored than they are about being stigmatised.

Remember the principles for commissioning which we learnt from looking at the case of gonorrhoea:

- data and research have to be made public
- information has to be widely disseminated and discussed within the communities affected
- the sexual behaviour which leads to STDs has to be made explicit (thankfully it is some time since we have seen coy terms used about transmission through 'bodily fluids'!)
- campaigns and programmes must be developed with (and we mean with, not for) the communities affected.

These can and should be more generally applied in order to reduce gonorrhoea incidence among all men and not just gay men. But it is the last of these principles which we feel is most likely to be 'missed' in commissioning for any target group such as men. It is here that the valuable insights into male socialisation provided elsewhere in this book provide commissioners (and those influencing commissioners) with the means with which to realise achievable outcomes – in sexual health as in any other area.

References

Department of Health 1992 The health of the nation. HMSO, London

Part 2
Developing practice

As we pointed out in Part 1, men's health work is still in its infancy in this country. Practice that has developed has tended to be sporadic and often initiated by individuals without the backing of a strategic overview. In Part 2 we have gathered examples of practice which illustrate not only the growing concern with men's health but also the thoughtfulness and willingness to experiment which is pushing the work onto the agenda of health authorities and Government. The contributions here come from practitioners and others with an overview of the issues. They show the potential that exists for developing work with different groups of men, for different conditions or health issues, in different settings and in different ways.

4

Men's health: what should health promotion units do?

Alec Kendall

This chapter covers:

- a conceptual base for the promotion of men's health
- a variation in health?
- narrowing the gap
- health promotion interventions at a local level
- key issues for practitioners
- practical pointers.

Introduction

Writing a chapter of some permanence at a time when the context for specialist health promotion services is subject to more or less continuous revision is a task that calls for caution. The places that health promotion specialists can call 'home' are many, and they now include work inside Primary Care Groups (PCGs) and Primary Care Trusts. There are diverse roles, too: some health promotion specialists will work on operational issues in the field; for others, strategic responsibilities in health and local authorities beckon in the world of the 'new' public health. This chapter does not examine the organisational structures we have become accustomed to recognise as health promotion units, but rather the planning framework that health promotion and public health professionals could use to secure health improvement for men.

The continued relative decline in the health and achievement of men does not call for a cautious response. On the contrary, a determined effort is needed by health promotion professionals wherever they may work to narrow the gender gap.

Work to promote the health of men in the 21st century can be seen in the light of the issues set out in Box 4.1. The interplay of opportunity and organisational change (Secretary of State for Health 1997) amply shows that there is not and never will be a single track to health improvement for people in general, and men in particular.

Box 4.1   Some 21st century health issues and their implications for the promotion of men's health

Modernising the NHS

We need to recognise the impacts on and opportunities for change in the field of men's health created by the emergence of *Health Improvement Programmes* (HImPs) and *Primary Care Groups/Trusts.*

The inclusive, partnership-based, developmental approach of HImPs offers the best chance we have of mainstreaming male health issues strategically and locally. The HImP process also enables us to consider identifying and developing a prime mover outside the NHS, where this would be more effective. The emphasis on reducing inequities in health at a local level is important to men's health work, especially if the HImP is being developed in the context of a *Health Action Zone* or *Healthy Living Centre* movement.

Primary Care Groups can facilitate the delivery of locality-based men's health promotion work, particularly where this has been prioritised in the HImP. With local representation and local commissioning, opportunities for effective joint action should multiply. The risk for specialised programmes for men in this environment is that effort and resources may be dispersed across several centres unless performance management systems have been fully deployed by Health Authorities. *Clinical Governance* and *Best Value* structures offer excellent opportunities for developing quality frameworks.

Health promotion: whose territory?

There is an active debate – whether it is a healthy one is open to conjecture – about the interface between health promotion specialists and the broad family of public health professions.

Box 4.1   Cont'd

One view is that public health approaches to improving the health of men could be critical to achieving support for releasing resources and gaining ownership of the issue at a local level. Professional territoriality at the public health/health promotion/public health nursing boundaries has the potential to divide and diminish this effort. A common framework for action is vital.

Specialist versus generalist

Some specialist health promotion services have created a locality structure for delivering their work. This has often been in response to the need to develop local expertise and services equitably across a wide geographical area. Locality health promotion staff need to adopt a generic role, but operationally this is twinned with a professional specialty. This enables effective skill-sharing and networking to take place across localities, but there are clear training implications for support from generic staff (for example, those based in PCGs) in the area of promoting men's health.

A conceptual base for the promotion of men's health

Few health promotion specialists will find difficulty modelling a theoretical base for their work. The real debate will focus on the appropriateness or effectiveness of the chosen perspective in planning their processes.

Critically now, as health promotion professionals take their proper place in the creation of national and local effectiveness measures, planning health promotion for men must take account of robust measures of success. Learmonth's discussion paper on these issues (Learmonth 1997) adapts Beattie's 1991 four-paradigm model to locate health promotion strategies and links them systematically to proposed measures of health gain. Of special note is Learmonth's annotation of the *Collective-Negotiated paradigm*: developing and auditing partnerships for health and promoting the use of research methods like Participatory Rapid Appraisal will ensure that community participation in needs assessment and priority-setting will be at the core of effective work with men.

Mapping and organising the work of health promotion specialists in the field of men's health also requires an appropriate framework. Merely designing programmes and processes to operate in parallel with those developed to promote women's health will not deliver the results we need to tackle a pervasive 'variation in health'.

A variation in health?

Without doubt, the current health status of men in this country represents all that is characteristic of a long-term, worsening inequity:

- Life expectancy at birth is 6 years greater for women than for men.

- Up to age 65, men have a three-and-a-half times higher risk of death from coronary heart disease than women.

- Loss of a job will double a middle-aged man's risk of dying within the next 5 years (Department of Health 1998).

- Young men are over-represented in the criminal justice system.

- Suicides among young men rose dramatically over the decade to 1998, against a fall in rates among women (Department of Health 1998).

- Antisocial behaviour in boys (five-sixths of the total of children with behavioural problems) is related negatively to intelligence; in girls it is positively associated (Bailey 1997).

- Boys make up 66% of children with learning difficulties.

- Boys under 5 are at greater risk of death from accidents than girls of the same age.

- The risk of accidental death for boys from the lowest social class is multiplied a further five times when compared with death rates in the highest social class (Department of Health 1998).

Given these facts, health promotion professionals determined to promote men's health could usefully consider using an 'inequalities' framework to plan and assess their work.

Table 4.1 **Two of the 'Closing the Gap' indicators for Birmingham, selected for their relevance to improving male health (Wood 1995)**

Indicator	Effective interventions in which health promotion plays a key role
Young male suicide (25–44)	■ Changing the design of car exhausts ■ Outreach youth services ■ Care Programme Approach ■ Detection and treatment of depression in primary care ■ Parenting skill assessments and recognition of behavioural disturbance ■ Appropriate services for young people with mental health problems
Death from coronary heart disease in middle age (45–64)	■ Increased taxation on tobacco ■ Opportunistic smoking cessation advice and follow-up in general practice ■ Targeting of men from ethnic minority groups where smoking rates are high

Narrowing the gap

In her 1995 Annual Report, the Director of Public Health for Birmingham identified 10 key indicators of the health of the local population (Wood 1995). These represented the most significant inequalities that could be detected and measured systematically in neighbourhoods across the city. As can be seen in Table 4.1, they were also linked to a range of effective interventions: one indicator referred specifically to the mental health of young men; another, relating to coronary heart disease, is not gender-specific but represents an area where the mortality risk is significantly higher for men.

Narrowing the health gap for men is dependent on developing sound methods of needs assessment and using epidemiological methods that are linked to clear and robust indicators of progress. Health promotion staff working closely with public health colleagues can place such benchmarks in the Health Improvement Programme (HImP) for their localities – perhaps the most important signal of commitment to the issue.

But effective needs assessment extends beyond epidemiology. Health promotion professionals use a wide range of tools in assessing need. Much of the work around the health of gay men, for example, has been remarkably successful in its targeting and research outcomes. Outreach work, one-to-one interviews and the use of anonymised questionnaires have informed work to provide effective health promotion and accessible services. Whether this level of success is routinely achieved in other areas of men's health is open to question.

The use of tools like rapid appraisals in local communities requires a special effort to be made to ensure that men are fully represented in the sampling process. Successive rapid appraisals on housing estates in Worcestershire have become more effective in obtaining the views of men to determine local health priorities (Department of Public Health 1996, 1998), but access has been principally through group interviews in local pubs and contacts with residents' associations. Job clubs, centres for the unemployed, foyer schemes, workplaces and – for young men particularly – youth outreach programmes and the internet all provide additional opportunities for rapid appraisal contact with men. The potential of this approach to set health work with men in the context of expressed need should be exploited to the full.

There remain too few access points to develop men's health issues. While health professionals are aware of the importance of the mass media, specialist interest magazines, partners and to a lesser extent friends, in reaching men (Holland, Mauthner and Sharpe 1996), it is the local or neighbourhood perspective that is likely to yield key entry points for effective work.

Health promotion interventions at a local level

Whitehead has reviewed evaluated interventions that aim to reduce inequalities in health (Whitehead 1995). She describes them as following into four groups of strategies, which:

- strengthen individuals (Level 1)
- strengthen communities (Level 2)
- improve access to services (Level 3)
- encourage economic and cultural change (Level 4).

Reviews carried out for the Dutch government, quoted by Whitehead, indicate that the most effective work to tackle inequalities in health involves strengthening the individual through the provision of information and personal support. There is every reason to believe that initiatives to improve the health of men in the UK should focus efforts in these areas, but unless cultural shifts in the arena of policy formulation are achieved, diversion of resources to effect change is unlikely to happen.

Table 4.2 maps some of the work in an inequalities framework that could be undertaken within a HImP for men. The list is not exhaustive but it takes advantage of the modernising agenda for the health and social services.

Conclusion

Public health and health promotion professionals working in the NHS family, local authorities and the non-statutory sector will continue to play a central role in securing and improving the health of men. Primary Care Group partnerships with social services professionals, and the joint investment planning process have created new and exciting opportunities to mainstream men's health across organisational boundaries. Health promoters are adept change agents, wherever they are employed, and nowhere is change so overdue as in the development of sustained improvement in the health of all men.

References

Bailey S 1997 Sadistic and violent acts in the young. Child Psychology and Psychiatry Review 2(3):93–94

Department of Health 1998 Our healthier nation. Department of Health, London

Department of Public Health 1996 The Warndon project. Worcestershire Health Authority, Worcester

Department of Public Health 1998 Westlands and your health. Worcestershire Health Authority, Worcester

Holland J, Mauthner M, Sharpe S 1996 Communicating health messages in the family. Health Education Authority, London

Learmonth A 1997 Health gain, effectiveness and health promotion. In: SHEPS Debate, special issue 1, Society of Health Education and Health Promotion Specialists, Glasgow

Table 4.2 Potential health improvement activity mapped by level and function

Function/Level	Strengthen individuals	Strengthen communities	Improve access to services	Encourage economic and social change
Training	■ Male health mentoring schemes ■ Lay health workers	■ Community development training for health and social care workers	■ Training for service providers on male health issues ■ Training in needs assessment	■ Training in credit union development ■ Joint training with LEA on the learning environment for boys in school
Policy development	■ Improve workplace health and personnel policies to promote a greater sense of job control among lower-grade working men	■ Regeneration programmes, Health Action Zones, Healthy Living Centres, Education Action Zones and HimPs that recognise inequalities in male health and achievement	■ Use Best Value reviews to ensure appropriateness of services to needs of men ■ Policy of benchmarking for men's health in NHS provision	■ Auditing policy work in the business sector for sensitivity to the special needs of men
Primary Care Group development	■ Maintain contact with young men in general practice in post-school years, and support through transitions ■ Provide gateways to local personal counselling and advice services like NHS Direct	■ Support training in public health nursing that recognises the effectiveness of community development approaches ■ Development of 'weak tie' networks to enhance job opportunities for unemployed men (Perri 6 1997)	■ Develop outreach primary care services in communities and workplaces ■ Support for community transport schemes and preparation for retirement courses	■ Clinical effectiveness work to extend the field of expertise in male health interventions ■ Support community safety partnerships in focusing on youth crime, diversionary approaches and parenting skills work

Key issues for practitioners

- There is real value for health promotion units in using an 'inequalities' framework to plan and assess their work with men.
- Clear methods of needs assessment and epidemiological approaches with a definite link to indicators of progress are crucial in promoting men's health.
- Health promotion professionals need to work closely with public health colleagues to ensure such indicators are incorporated in implementation plans at all tiers.

Practical pointers

- Needs assessment should encompass more than just epidemiology. Other tools such as outreach work, one-to-one interviews, anonymous questionnaires and rapid appraisal have been shown to work with groups of gay men, and could be widened to be used with men generally, if an effort is made to include men in the sampling process.
- The local or neighbourhood perspectives are the most likely sources of entry points for health promotion work with men.

Perri 6 1997 Escaping poverty. Demos, London

Secretary of State for Health 1997 The new NHS. HMSO, London

Whitehead M 1995 Tackling inequalities: a review of policy initiatives. In: Benzeval M, Judge K, Whitehead M (eds) Tackling inequalities in health. King's Fund, London

Wood A (ed) 1995 Closing the gap: ten benchmarks for equity and quality in health. Birmingham Health Authority, Birmingham

5

The development of men's health in Australia

Richard Fletcher

Introduction

At the end of 1997 a survey was circulated to all health regions in New South Wales (NSW) in Australia asking them to identify existing men's health services. It was to be used by the Men's Health Advisory Group, a task force set up by the NSW Health Minister, to develop a men's health strategy. This survey was a significant event in the development of men's health in Australia. The covering letter from the Director General of Health made it clear that the survey was a priority, marking the arrival of men's health as the ordinary business of the health services. However, the survey also revealed the uncertainty surrounding what constitutes 'men's health'. It was felt necessary to spell out a definition of men's health and of a men's health service.

Men's health

A men's health issue is a disease or condition unique to men, more prevalent in men, more serious among men, for which risk factors are different for men or for which different interventions are required for men. This definition of men's health paraphrases the United States Public Health Service Action Plan for Women's Health (1991) definition of women's health, and was adopted by the NSW Men's Health Advisory Group without comment. The Men's Health Service definition, however, required considerable discussion, because it was recognised that asking many health service managers 'What are you currently offering in men's health?' would elicit the (puzzled) response 'Well ... everything. Except for specific women's health services, all our services are open to men, many of them see mostly men.'

The definition of Men's Health Services arrived at for the purposes of the survey was as follows. Men's Health Services are those which:

■ address men's health issues
■ pay particular attention to targeting males, engaging males or treating males
■ incorporate an acknowledgement that existing services, whatever their merits, require a fresh approach to males' health in order to improve males' health status.

This definition was an attempt to force health managers to consider the central claim of men's health, that simply targeting males, or having males deliver health services, was not sufficient to ensure that males' needs were recognised and addressed. As was to be expected, many managers took up the challenge, while others simply reported 'no specific services'.

The fact that the survey took place at such a senior level is testimony to the persistence of the notion that 'something must be done' about men's health. The clumsiness of the definition however, and the need in a survey to try to dramatically change the perspective of senior management is revealing of how large a barrier exists to the promotion of men's health. These two factors – the insistent evidence of the need for men's health to be addressed, and the confusion about just what is needed – underlie the uneven policy development process in men's health in Australia (and the chaotic arrangements for emerging service delivery and health promotion to men).

The first major health policy initiatives began in South Australia, and at a national level in 1995. In August of that year the then Commonwealth Health Minister in the Labour Government launched the National Men's Health Conference and pledged to develop a national policy. She also hinted that substantial funding would follow. This brought a good deal of media interest, including features over several days on the state of men's health. Over the next few months the Commonwealth initiated a preliminary consultation process with key stakeholders in each state, and a draft policy was produced which called for an extensive consultation with health services, consumers and interest groups. Men began to appear as a target category for other health funding bodies. When the Labour Government was replaced with a Conservative/Liberal National party coalition in 1997, the new Minister cancelled the men's health policy process. Other Government bodies took heed and men's health as a legitimate funding category began to disappear again.

State policies however have continued to develop. In Western Australia (where the only university to offer men's health courses is located) a Men's Health Policy was released in November 1997 at the Second National Men's Health Conference by the Liberal Health Minister. The conference attracted many delegates, including a large contingent of Aboriginal representatives. A draft Western Australia Aboriginal Men's Health Policy was also released. In NSW a men's health strategy process was initiated by the Labour Health Minister. In 1998 a discussion paper entitled *Strategic directions in men's health* was released, followed by the launch, in July 1999, of *Moving forward in men's health*. Although this document nominated a range of strategies, including a grants programme for innovations, work with general practitioners and developing appropriate resources for men, only the Men's Health and Information and Resource Centre was actually funded, with a 3-year grant.

Programme developments

The difficulty in articulating men's health for policy development has its parallel in the delivery of health services. The main obstacle in developing men's health programmes has not been opposition from those suggesting that men should not have good health, but from those assuming that men are already taken care of by existing services. An associated belief is that men are incapable of change. For example, a frequent response to the clear statistical evidence of higher male mortality are statements such as: 'Well yes, the figures are not too good, but men don't care about their health; they won't go to the doctor and they are too macho to admit that they have a problem'.

This view of men and the mechanisms of social change have influenced the public understanding of men's health activity in Australia. Because women's health was so clearly a part of the women's movement – a widespread social movement advocating radical change in the way society and social institutions treated women – it has been assumed that men's health would evolve in a like fashion. Since men have not taken to the streets it is concluded either that there is no problem or that men won't change anyway. A corollary of this view is that there is a necessary antagonism between men's health and women's health. This misunderstanding is reinforced by media reports of the 'men's movement'. The men's movement activity which appears to be most recognisable to the media (and to many left-wing commentators) is made up of groups who, mimicking the consciousness-raising groups of the early women's liberation movement, meet in all-male groups to discuss their grievances and link their feelings of injustice to social practices. While some Fathers' Rights groups approximate this model, there is no evidence that the majority of men's groups are based on notions of injustice or see women's power as the source of their problems. More importantly, the activity of men's groups has had little direct impact on the development of men's health programmes. In fact, it is female nurses who have initiated many of the 'men's health' programmes now available. The Men's Health Night, for example, was pioneered by a rural community health nurse concerned about the poor health status of men in her area. The model has been adapted to other regional and metropolitan areas.

Men's Health Nights

Men's Health Nights were initially held in rural towns across central Victoria during 1996 and early 1997. The format in each case was to have local medical practitioners and well-known sports personalities speak about the health situation for men in a male-friendly environment such as a football or rugby club. Advertising brochures were distributed through local networks including men's service clubs, offering a prize of a 'romantic weekend' for two to be drawn on the night.

In monthly follow-up sessions, general practitioners talked about cardiovascular disease, cancer, stress and prostate problems. The participants were screened for high blood pressure, plasma cholesterol, glucose, as well as their height and weight being recorded. Following the success of these forums, similar events have been initiated in other rural centres and capital cities across Australia.

Such programmes are based on alliances between traditional healthcare providers. While the participants and organisers (often female nurses or health promotion officers) are aware of the discussion about men's changing roles, they have few formal links with 'men's groups'. Where men's health activities have sprung directly from groups readily identified as part of a 'men's movement', their focus has been on the broader social aspects of health.

Men's Help Line

The Men's Help Line originated at a men's festival in 1994 in Brisbane. The four men attending a meeting there each contributed $200 and the line was in the telephone directory. At that time there was no men's classification in the community service pages of the phone book. Callers have to find the number in the phone book under Men. In 1996 the line was taking 10 calls a day. No advertising has been done as it is thought this would overload the resources of the group.

Approximately half the calls received are about relationship breakdowns. 8% are men's movement calls – wanting to find a men's group, information about the men's festival and so on. Another 8% are from professionals – social workers, doctors, counsellors etc. One doctor rang the service and said: 'I've got this guy here who's been raped. He went to the rape crisis centre and was told they don't deal with men. Where can I refer him?'

Besides those working at the community level and health professionals, health organisations have also helped to draw attention to men's health. Merck Sharp and Dohme, a major pharmaceutical company, has promoted men's conferences, produced books on men's health and assisted in the formation of the Prostate Disease Awareness Committee, which involves peak health and 'male' community bodies in raising the profile of men's health, particularly prostate disease. Pharmacists' organisations have also instigated men's health services.

The Prostate Health Information Line

The Prostate Health Information Line was set up in 1994 with an educational grant from industry as part of the Pharmacy Self Care programme. This is a subscription service of the Program of the Pharmaceutical Society of Australia, which has approximately 1400 subscribers (pharmacies).

The line took approximately 2000 calls in its first 20 months. Around 15–20% of callers are female, and more than 95% of calls come from the public. The purpose of the line is not to diagnose – that would be inappropriate, not to say impossible. Instead, callers ring with a particular query, or simply to find out about possible symptoms of prostate disease, so they know what to look out for. Callers frequently comment that they appreciate having the time to discuss their concerns. It would seem that in the doctor's surgery people are reluctant to ask their questions, or if they do there is insufficient time to receive adequate answers. In some ways the Prostate Health Information Line serves as a conduit between patients and their physician, as every caller is encouraged to consult with his general practitioner or specialist.

Heart health assessment days

Heart disease is frequently cited as a major cause of death for men, and men's heart attacks have been highlighted in the public perception of health risk for many years. The Australian National Heart Foundation, launched in the 1950s, is a pre-eminent health organisation, a source of expertise and a leading site for heart-related research and health promotion. Like many other prominent health bodies, it has been reluctant to address men's health as a new issue (as defined in the NSW survey above) as part of its activities. However, some community-based health workers have used the widespread acceptance of heart health screening to engage men in a wider range of health prevention activities.

Evidence of males' poor heart health and poor attendance at health centres in general led, in 1995, to a project being set up in a rural New South Wales health district to screen males for heart health. An important part of the strategy was to conduct the sessions in the small towns (populations of 300) surrounding the regional centre. As part of the screening, men were asked about their priorities for health information.

The lead-up to the sessions involved considerable preparation by the Heart Health Team, including discussions with male organisations and well-known men in each town. The team was unusual in that it consisted of a female health educator and a male rural counsellor who had previously been a farrier. This combination gave them entry to many areas of the rural societies where the assessments were to be held.

Of the men screened, 80% were either farmers or labourers. A follow-up phone survey revealed behaviour change in a significant proportion of them in the areas of diet, exercise levels, alcohol consumption and smoking habits. Other health issues identified by the men themselves were:

- farm-based chemicals
- stress and stress management
- cancer.

Pre-op education for radical prostatectomy

Improving men's health is often taken to mean health promotion, or at least attention to the major killers such as heart disease. And it is frequently assumed that men's 'macho' attitudes or beliefs make up much of the problem. In the case of men undergoing radical prostatectomy, however, it has been shown that major improvements can be made by changing the treatment of men within the healthcare system.

In 1994 a clinical nurse consultant in urology at Royal Newcastle Hospital (NSW) noticed a number of men arriving at the Incontinence Clinic after prostate surgery who were angry about their symptoms of incontinence, retrograde ejaculation and impotence. She observed that many had purchased inappropriate aids and that they lacked basic information about their conditions. Many also had been in difficulty for some time and had found out about the clinic only by accident. A number felt that they had not been informed of the impact of likely side-effects of the surgery. While she realised that their claims that the general practitioners and urologists had not discussed these issues with them were untrue, they clearly had not understood what 'a little bit of leakage' could mean in daily living. She contacted the urologists practising in the area and offered to set up a pre-op education service. The service has been operating since late 1994.

Men referred to the unit are first sent printed information. They then attend a 1-hour introductory talk where they are shown the equipment to be used, such as catheters, and discuss the operation, hospital procedures and the likely effects of the operation. They come back 1 week before the operation to review their understanding, and they are seen again after the operation. They may call the clinic at any time. Reports from men attending indicate that their experience of surgery is less traumatic and their use of aids for subsequent conditions is more appropriate.

Gutbusters waist loss programme for men

It was long assumed by health promotion professionals that men would not be interested in losing weight. Focus group research among steelworkers found that not only did they want to lose weight, but they had definite ideas about what sort of weight loss course would suit men. Using this information, the Gutbusters waist loss programme was designed, and it was different to traditional diet-based approaches to weight loss.

The programme started up in 1991. Key factors were:

- it was a male-only course
- advertising stressed males with big bellies
- there was an information-based teaching style using lifestyle change based on fat balance rather than diet.

The numbers of men completing the basic course (more than 40 000 in the first 3 years) make it the largest weight loss course for men anywhere in the world. Initial results reported in scientific journals (e.g. *International Journal of Obesity* 1996) are encouraging. The programme, under the name Gutbusters, has since been sold to Heinz.

Noongar men's health manual

Aboriginal men have a life expectancy up to 20 years below that of nonindigenous men. Indigenous organisations in

Western Australia and Queensland were amongst the first community groups to call for attention to be paid to the issue of men's health.

The Noongar (Aboriginal) men of Western Australia have developed a comprehensive men's health manual with step-by-step guides for group discussions of the following issues:

- becoming powerful
- men's roles and responsibilities
- family violence
- abuse
- grief
- trauma and depression
- substance abuse

The starting points for taking action are listed as:

- recognising that the loss of men's roles is a problem
- accepting responsibility for reestablishing men's roles in the family and community
- recognising how our past has hurt all Noongar people
- seeking family or community help and support
- developing men's activities
- recognising that Wadjelas (nonindigenous people) don't understand our people
- developing community roles that will give our young men the guidance they need to survive and prosper in today's world.

Conclusion

While the examples discussed in this chapter are not representative of all men's health services in Australia, they are illustrative of some important trends. The disparate collection of individual and organisational initiatives presented here is not underpinned by a unified conception of men's health, or by a single theoretical, ideological or professional position. They have developed with limited resources (except for the pharmaceutical industry programmes) and in the face of indifference from health and medical authorities. This has made it difficult to translate the efforts of innovators into supportive policies, but it has also ensured that fluctuating political commitment to men's health has not halted the momentum for addressing men's health needs in practice.

Key issues for practitioners

- The experience from Australia suggests that difficulty in articulating what 'men's health' and a men's health 'service' are is a real barrier to the development of policy. Simply targeting males or having men deliver health services is not sufficient to ensure men's health needs are recognised and addressed.

- Other key obstacles to developing men's health programmes follow from the belief that men are already taken care of by existing services and that men are incapable of change.

- It has often been assumed that there is a conflict between men's health and women's health, but in fact health programmes for men have often been initiated by women.

Practical pointers

- Health information telephone helplines aimed at men are well used by men (and women).

- Taking services to where men already are, e.g. heart health screening programmes in small communities for specific groups of men, gets a higher take-up than expecting men to attend existing services.

6

It Takes Two: a contraceptive campaign aimed at men

Lorraine Hoare and Joan Walsh

This chapter covers:

- designing *It Takes Two: creating opportunities for clients*
- research
- professional practice
- men's approaches to contraceptive responsibility
- research into practice: a framework for practice development
- designing and disseminating resources
- proactive media work
- interactive dissemination
- evaluation
- key issues for practitioners
- practical pointers.

Introduction

This chapter describes an initiative which explored men's approaches to contraceptive use and responsibility, researched professional practice, identified practical ways of including men in contraceptive service provision and promoted coverage of men and contraception in the media. The work was undertaken by the Contraceptive Education Service (CES), which is funded by the Department of Health, and provided in partnership by the Health Education Authority and the Family Planning Association.

Designing *It Takes Two: creating opportunities for clients*

As part of its work, the CES has a commitment to targeted contraceptive health promotion work with different population groups, including men. A major initiative called *It Takes Two* was launched in 1997, with the aim of bridging a gap – supporting health professionals in creating opportunities for clients to discuss contraceptive needs and concerns, and encouraging men to ask health professionals for contraceptive information and advice. It was decided that the initiative should:

- reflect existing knowledge about the impact of men's socialisation and its impact on men's use of health services (Davidson & Lloyd 1995)
- target men directly as individuals in order to be effective in reaching heterosexually active men
- reach those most likely to be receptive to 'sex and your health' messages (e.g. those with immediate concerns about unintended paternity and/or sexually transmitted infection)
- be designed and developed in a way which secured the involvement and ongoing support of health professionals, and which encouraged sharing of professional learning and skills across different healthcare settings and between different professional disciplines.

The difficulties of targeting men and encouraging their inclusion in sexual health promotion were not underestimated. Attempting to raise awareness of one aspect of health within a social and cultural framework where expectations of men's interest in general were low would inevitably be an uphill struggle. In addition, we wished to challenge the existing social expectations and attitudes relating to men, not only as users of health services, but also as key commissioners, designers and providers of those services. The initiative would be at best a starting point, and would inevitably highlight barriers as well as opportunities. There would be resistance to an approach whose success depended on staff looking to encourage communication by and with men on sensitive topics in an already overstretched service, where prevention and health promotion work may in any case be undervalued and under-resourced.

Having reviewed uptake of primary and secondary health-care services by men, it was decided to focus on genitourinary medicine (GUM) and sexual health clinics in the first instance. Only a small proportion of heterosexually active men use these services, but it was considered that they were those most likely to be receptive to a contraceptive health promotion message. Another important consideration was professional expertise. GUM/sexual health practitioners have substantially more experience of working with men on sexual health issues than other primary care professionals, so this approach offered the greatest opportunities for cross-boundary dissemination of learning and skills.

Research

Professional practice
CES commissioned research to identify possible points of intervention, looking in particular at whether, when and how health professionals in general practice, family planning clinics and GUM/sexual health clinics report discussing contraception with men and women.

With regard to differences in consultations with men and women, the research findings confirmed expectations. Most of the health professionals interviewed said that they provided contraceptive services only or mostly to women, and all reported being less likely to discuss contraception and, in particular, to initiate discussion of contraception, with men than with women. Observational research found that only 5% of contraceptive materials on display in waiting rooms could be regarded as targeting men.

Men's approaches to contraceptive responsibility
During focus group work with men (covering contraceptive responsibility, condom use, decision-making, responsibility and communication with sexual partners) three different approaches to contraceptive responsibility emerged:

1. opportunistic
2. passive
3. prepared.

Men who usually adopted the 'opportunistic' approach:

■ had internalised the risks and consequences of unprotected sex – they were aware of the risks, and aware that the consequences for them were real and undesirable
■ recognised a responsibility to protect partners' health and wellbeing, as well as their own
■ but approached contraceptive responsibility and condom use inconsistently, depending on the particular circumstances of each encounter
■ lacked confidence in carrying condoms or in discussing contraception and condom use with partners
■ were sometimes prepared to take the initiative in mentioning condom use – if the situation was perceived as risky, or to impress or persuade a potential partner
■ abandoned condom use at the first opportunity.

The 'passive' approach was characterised by:

■ feeling remote and removed from the risks and consequences of unprotected sex, preferring not to think about them
■ being sometimes motivated to use condoms as self-protection but very rarely raising the issue of contraception or condom use (unless, for example, a new partner was perceived as being particularly 'risky')
■ using condoms reluctantly, e.g. if a partner asked or insisted
■ lacking the confidence to discuss contraception, and feeling unwilling and/or unable to take the initiative.

Men adopting the 'prepared' approach:

■ had a strong sense and realistic understanding of the consequences of unprotected sex for themselves
■ were well-motivated to use condoms routinely, to protect themselves and their partners
■ were confident in carrying, discussing and using condoms as a matter of course, and reported proactively discussing condom use with partners
■ had a strong initial sense of shared responsibility for contraception – but this declined when condom use was abandoned as trust was established and the sense of risk decreased (after Health Education Authority 1997).

These categories are not categories of men, but categories of approach. Generally speaking, most men's approach to contraceptive responsibility (and safer sex) tends towards the 'opportunistic'. It is situational and based on one-off judgments about the particular circumstances of an encounter.

The key point to emerge from the research is that men can and do move between the different approaches outlined above. This means that health professionals can have an impact by:

- motivating men to develop a more consistent 'prepared' approach
- informing, advising and supporting men to devise and implement personal risk-reduction strategies.

It also follows that:

- Promoting a consistent approach to contraception among men in the (majority) 'opportunistic' group means enabling them to translate theory into practice, and to strengthen their role in the decision-making process.

- Promoting contraceptive responsibility among men with a 'passive' approach means raising awareness of the risks associated with the 'ostrich position' and encouraging a sense of self-preservation.

- Supporting contraceptive use by 'prepared' men means sustaining motivation and a sense of shared responsibility for contraception in longer-term relationships.

Research into practice: a framework for practice development

The key findings of the research were discussed in meetings with a multidisciplinary Advisory Group of GUM/sexual health professionals to:

- determine the implications for professional practice
- explore the feasibility and practicality of different options for the initiative
- develop materials for dissemination.

In the course of work with the Advisory Group, it became apparent that medical and sexual history taking was a key process, representing a good point of intervention for the CES initiative. History-taking forms and pro-formas are very influential in that they structure the professional in terms of client dialogue, determining in advance which subjects will be raised and which will not be mentioned unless the client takes the lead. Forms are used to record information, but also serve to legitimise question areas – 'I just have to complete this form' – making it clear that the professional is not making judgements about the individual client. The message is clear: 'we ask everybody this'.

Men and women are generally asked different questions, because of obvious biological differences, but also reflecting the cultural beliefs and expectations of the health professionals, such as:

■ 'Men aren't interested in contraception – they don't get pregnant.'

■ 'Why ask men about contraception when there isn't a pill for men?'

■ 'You can't ask men about paternities – they wouldn't know.'

When taking a medical or sexual history from a woman, there are a number of points at which it is obviously legitimate, from the client and the professional perspective, for the subject of contraception to be raised. There is a logical place for a question about contraception – somewhere amongst questions about menarche, menstruation, relationship status, pregnancy history, pregnancy outcomes and intentions. Regardless of their circumstances, women of reproductive age expect to be asked about pregnancies and contraceptive use, in just about any medical consultation. Both are regarded as relevant and important items of information in women's healthcare.

In contrast, while taking a traditional history from men there are generally no obvious opportunities for initiating discussion about:

■ previous paternities
■ pregnancy outcomes
■ contraceptive use
■ pregnancy/paternity intentions.

Men do not expect to be asked about contraception and paternity, which of course makes it harder for professionals to do so. Having had little practice, men are not fluent in 'contraceptive-speak', so they are very unlikely to take the initiative in discussing contraceptive needs and concerns, let alone unintended paternity, when the subjects are clearly not on the professional agenda.

This circular situation can only serve to reinforce professional beliefs about men not being interested in contraception, and cultural stereotypes about contraception not being a subject of relevance to 'real' men. Though pertinent to men's health and healthcare, questions about contraception and paternity may never be asked. Men are, in effect, often excluded from the 'contraceptive culture' and from contraceptive services by a self-perpetuating process.

The *It Takes Two: creating opportunities for clients* intervention sought to address this problem by promoting dialogue between health professionals and heterosexually active men. The principal message was: take the initiative and create opportunities for discussion – don't wait for the other person to ask.

Key concerns which emerged from the Advisory Group meeting were that:

- The group of men targeted might, quite reasonably, want to focus exclusively on the original reason for attending a clinic (i.e. concern that they have/may have a sexually transmitted infection).

- Any frameworks/suggestions for practice development would have to take into account the very considerable constraints on time and other resources in clinical practice.

- Given the wealth of materials targeting gay men, resources distributed for public display in a GUM/sexual health setting would have to be very distinctive in order to reach heterosexually active men effectively, whilst also being acceptable to staff working in the clinic.

Designing and disseminating resources

The *It Takes Two: creating opportunities for clients* pack was distributed in February 1997 to Health Advisors and Senior Nurses in GUM/sexual health clinics in England. It contained:

- Summaries of research conducted with professionals and with men.

- Two motivational posters for display, one targeting men and women (with the message 'You can ask a doctor or nurse at this clinic about contraception') and one specifically aimed at men with an 'opportunistic' approach to contraceptive use (with the message 'Men ask here for contraceptive information and advice').

- Credit-card-style leaflets promoting the CES information and telephone helpline service, with a display dispenser.

- The CES leaflet *Your guide to contraception* and the newly available HEA leaflet *The condom guide*.

- a suggested framework for developing practice (which grew out of the research findings), focusing on sexual history taking and the discussion of contraception (see Box 6.1).

Proactive media work

From February 1997 the *It Takes Two* materials were distributed to 200 daily and weekly newspapers and magazines. Collaborative work with media representatives ensured positive coverage of the initiative, with longer features appearing in both professional and popular publications (e.g. *Nursing Times, Take a Break*). Media slots about and for men were paid for on Virgin Radio, and obtained free in the form of 58 local radio interviews lasting between 30 seconds and 5 minutes. This work was undertaken to support direct dissemination work with professionals.

Interactive dissemination

It Takes Two was also disseminated at a series of half-day multidisciplinary seminars held in different locations in England, attended by professionals from the fields of family planning, GUM/sexual health and health promotion. They were offered further information about:

- research findings into the impact of men's socialisation on the use of health services
- successful approaches to working with men on sexual health issues
- the development of the *It Takes Two* materials.

Facilitated workshops were run to explore how the *It Takes Two* pack ideas and materials could be used and further

Box 6.1   The *It Takes Two* framework for developing practice (after Health Education Authority 1998)

Developing a consistent approach to sexual history taking and the discussion of contraception

Reviewing current practice

Review documentation. Look at the case notes of a sample of men and women who report being heterosexually active. Assess how clearly and consistently information is recorded about the clients':

- paternities or pregnancies
- attitudes to contraception and patterns of contraceptive use
- perceptions of the risk of unintended paternity/pregnancy and its implications
- personal strategy to reduce the risk of unintended paternity/ pregnancy.

What information was the client given about contraceptive methods and services?

Was condom use explained and demonstrated?

Use this information to evaluate current practice:

- Are all staff asking the same questions of all heterosexually active women and men?

- Are clients' responses being recorded consistently by different members of staff?

- If questions were not asked, is this clearly recorded and the reasons noted?

- Do the notes provide a complete and accessible 'contraceptive profile' of the client?

Moving forward: working to develop practice

If there are gaps or areas of inconsistency, work with colleagues to draft and agree a policy for the documentation of sexual history taking and guidelines for discussing contraception which will:

- Improve the quality and consistency of client care
- save time and improve communication between different staff members.

Box 6.1   Cont'd

Areas to look at (in single-discipline groups and as a team) include:

■ Existing policies and guidelines.

■ The purpose, wording and value of the questions asked during sexual history taking.

■ Ways of recording responses to open and closed questions about contraceptive use.

■ Ways of recording and/or summarising broader discussions about contraception.

■ Which clients, client groups and/or consultations should be targeted, taking into account the likelihood of loss to follow-up.

■ Ways of creating opportunities for men and women to raise contraceptive needs and concerns.

With regard to staff, subjects to consider might include:

■ Roles and responsibilities – who does what, when and with which client groups?

■ Communication between professionals – coordinating activities and making referrals.

■ Training – what training will different staff need, and who will provide it?

Discussion of practice could cover:

■ Monitoring practice development – who is responsible, what support do they need?

■ Auditing and evaluating changes in practice – who will do it, when, how and how often?

---

disseminated in participants' own professional settings and locales.

Seminar participants were asked to describe what support would be required at their local level to implement *It Takes Two*. Support at management level emerged as a key factor. Participants were also asked to consider what resources would be useful for the future and, in particular, what the CES could provide. Two resources were in demand at every seminar:

1. Contraceptive information materials designed specifically for men, which could be used as 'ice-breakers' during consultations to introduce the subject of contraception and which men could take away with them.
2. Training resources for professionals working with men.

These were subsequently developed and published by CES in 1998, in the form of a credit-card-style leaflet entitled *Men: this is for you*, and a series of training exercises called *It Takes Two training resource: sexual health, contraception and men*.

Evaluation

Informal feedback and formal evaluations suggested that three key features contributed to the success of *It Takes Two*:

1. The approach was highly innovative – it was men-friendly and positive throughout, rather than being 'finger-wagging' or 'guilt-tripping'.
2. The model of approaches to contraceptive responsibility (opportunistic, passive and prepared) offered a useful way in for practitioners both to understand men's attitudes and behaviours, and to work more constructively with male clients.
3. The suggestions for developing professional practice were regarded as being practical and realistic.

This last point is particularly significant: to have any credibility, developmental work with health professionals must be grounded in their day-to-day reality. Including men must be based on changing professional assumptions about men – about their level of interest and their need to be included. Approaches must be structured, consistent and persistent (Davidson & Lloyd 1995). Publications for men must be targeted at men directly, and be clearly 'for men'.

References

Davidson N, Lloyd T 1995 Working with heterosexual men on sexual health. Health Education Authority, London
Health Education Authority 1997 It Takes Two: creating opportunities for clients. Health Education Authority, London

Key issues for practitioners

- Given the lack of knowledge about men and health, research provides a useful base from which to design effective interventions with men and with health professionals.

- Men do not expect to be asked about contraception and paternity, making it harder for health professionals to approach these topics with them. This creates a vicious circle, in which men are effectively excluded from the contraceptive culture.

- Including men in contraceptive use needs to be based on changing professionals' assumptions about men, particularly about their level of interest.

Practical pointers

- A 'men-friendly' approach was critical to the success of this campaign.

- The model of approaches to contraceptive responsibility which emerged from the research was that men may move between 'opportunistic', 'passive' and 'prepared' stances.

- Interventions, for example the use of sexual history taking, need to be structured, consistent and persistent.

- Publications for men must be targeted directly at men.

Health Education Authority 1998 It Takes Two: creating opportunities for clients. Sexual health, contraception and men: a training resource. Health Education Authority, London

7

Developing resources

Paul Brown

Introduction

Having worked with young people since 1980, one of the biggest frustrations I have experienced is the lack of up-to-date, practical resources for developing positive initiatives with young men. Regardless of your experience, working with young men will often push you to the limits of both your patience and skills. The need to develop this area is clear, but often workers ask the question: How? Any tool that can help us to communicate with young men is to be welcomed. In this chapter we will look at developing different kinds of resources. Those described below were targeted at young men with the specific aim of supporting professional workers to:

- raise issues of health education
- encourage young men to talk
- increase their awareness and knowledge of health issues.

Resources for young men

There are various kinds of resources: books, videos, games, posters ... the list goes on. But none of these are any use if the necessary thinking about their appropriateness has not been done. Think about your audience carefully. It's no good making a video which gives all the right health education messages, if the young men you are working with cannot identify with the characters. In that case they will spend the time either 'taking the piss' out of the characters, or denying that the issue relates to them. So if you are working with young black men, for example, make sure there are black characters in the video.

It is also important to reflect real life scenarios that the young men can see themselves in. Think about the places you see young men hang out in, and try to reflect these. This will enable them to identify with the issue. Consider the content carefully too. Is it appropriate to the client group you are working with? One of the most used health education resources over the last 10 years is The Grapevine Game. However, when it was played with a group of young Asian men they raised real questions about the language used and the relevance of the game to their culture. Although it had been tried and tested over the years, this resource had clearly been developed with white British culture in mind, and there was no added information or guidelines for working with young people of other cultures.

When developing a health education resource for young men it is important that you consider a number of areas, such as young men's attitudes, awareness and feelings about the subject:

- How do the young men feel about talking about sex?

- How much information do they think they need?

- How embarrassed will they be if you ask them a question they can't answer?

A sure way to make your group work last only one session is to start asking young men questions that they either find embarrassing or don't think they know the answer to.
      Clarity is also important:

- Why are you doing the work?
- Is it your agenda, or your manager's, your funder's, or that of other members of staff?

Unless the young men you want to involve have some owner-ship of the project and have in some way instigated it, your starting point – and therefore your chances of success – will be greatly reduced.

Another consideration is the skills of the worker. At one level you can use any resource to develop the work, but the skills of the worker, that person's knowledge of and relationship with the group are significant factors. Also important if you want the young men to increase understanding and share experiences are:

- adequate preparation
- timing – don't set up the session at a time when the young men either want to watch football or a favourite television programme
- approach.

Safe video

Safe is a 24-minute video made by a group of professional workers all working with young men around health education issues. The video originated as a result of an assessment that there were limited resources in this area and that Danny's Big Night produced by the FPA in 1985 was the only recognised boys' work video available. The primary purpose of Safe was to raise issues of health education for young black men, as it was felt that there were very few resources that were appropriate to the educational needs of this group. Those that did exist were outdated and issue-focused rather than person-focused.

During the making of Safe it was important to ensure that we considered a number of factors in relation to the target audience. Some of these factors were straightforward, such as ensuring that the main characters were black. Others were not so clear cut. The think-ing behind the video was that it needed to target young black men, but in a subtle way that gave all the right health education messages without – like a lot of health education resources – being 'in your face'. We needed to get a balance between realism i.e. the settings that the video showed the characters in, and the health education issues.

It became very clear early on in the development stage of the script that the health education content (which had been researched) was not enough to engage the potential audience. It was essential that we also ensured the video reflected the kind of settings young black men could see themselves in, without marginalising them. Settings such as the gym, the barber's and the garage were all felt to be areas where young men would feel comfortable and able to see themselves in, and so would encourage communication.

It was also important to identify how young men communicate. Recognising that this is often the biggest single issue that stops young men from getting vital sources of information we felt we had to include banter and humour (both verbal and nonverbal). Vital too were choosing the right music, the right clothes and the right language. An example of how easy it is to get one of these things wrong came to light during the launch, where it was pointed out to us that the music we had used was 'East Coast Rap', which is an aggressive type of rap music associated with crime, and what we should have used was 'West Coast Rap', which is associated with communication and education.

Once the issues of settings and communication had been considered we felt there was a need to go back to the health education issues in order to identify how they could be reflected within the chosen settings and using the forms of communication that had been identified as appropriate for young men.

We felt there was a need to enable young men to use banter and humour when discussing serious health education issues, without those issues being seen as trivial and unimportant. There was also the need to create an environment or setting where a discussion about drugs or sex was not inappropriate and did not look out of place. So for example young men talking about condom use in a barber's would be seen as inappropriate, as it is a public environment, whereas having the same conversation in a garage while working on cars is OK, as this is a private environment.

 ## *Cut It Out* poster campaign

Posters and people are also types of resource that can be used to develop work with young men. An example of this was a project called

Cut It Out, a peer education project that looked at issues of teenage smoking and minority communities. The project involved training young men about the health education issues in relation to smoking. They had no smoking signs cut into their hair, which were then dyed different colours and photographed, to be turned into posters.

The idea to use the medium of hair as a focus for a health education project came from watching a *Black Britain* television programme which featured a local barber discussing the growing fashion of young black people and their various hair designs. We felt hair was something everyone could and would relate to.

Once we had decided to use hair as our focus the options in relation to health education were somewhat limited: did we look at issues of safe sex and condom use based on that well-known phrase 'Something for the weekend, Sir?', or did we consider another angle? The idea of addressing smoking came from the fact that the local health authority had anti-smoking targets based on research, and the barber, although allowing smoking in his shop, did not allow it while customers were in his chair.

In developing this project it was important to ensure that the young men we selected were clear about their role as peer educators and how they could best use the posters and related information. We had to consider how young people in schools and youth clubs would relate to these young men, and realised it was important that the young men we chose:

- were 'streetwise'
- had credibility in the local area
- were seen by young people as positive role models in the community.

The message the young men were relaying had to be consistent i.e. you have choices and these are the potential consequences of your choices.

The young men used three resources to develop the work:

1. posters
2. written information
3. themselves – both in terms of their knowledge and the message that was cut into their hair.

This project enabled us to develop young people as well as materials as effective resources.

Summary of guidelines for resource development

Dating and shelf life

Ageing is something you can do very little about but it needs to be a consideration when developing a resource. The things you do have control over, such as the dress of characters (in videos or posters) and the language used, must be as up-to-date as possible at launch. This will not only help sales and use, but also give the resource a longer shelf life.

Information is always changing, and people's attitudes are always developing. When researching your resource think in terms of a shelf life of 3–5 years. This will enable you to develop, market and launch your resource, and will also help with any form of evaluation you intend to carry out.

Target group

When developing your resource you must be clear about identifying your target group. You will then be able to consider effectively issues such as communication. It may be, for example, that to engage young men, visual communication is better than written communication. Using relevant, up-to-date issues that young men can relate to, such as dress, music, sport and body image, is a sure way of enabling your potential target group to show interest.

Language

There is often a thin line between using language that young men feel is real and language that is inappropriate for an educational resource. You will need to satisfy yourself that you have got the balance right between street slang and everyday language. Also, bear in mind regional and cultural language differences.

Research

Make sure you are clear about what is fact and what is fiction. During your research phase ensure that you have your client group in mind and that the information you are trying to share with them is up-to-date and relevant to their needs, rather than to yours or your funders'. You also need to be aware that the majority of information young men will have acquired about health issues may well have been either from male boasting or hearsay.

Once you have developed your resource, test it: you may be surprised at what you find. '*Safe*', for example, was aimed at young black men, but we found during the testing stage that it prompted young women to raise questions about their knowledge of the issues affecting young men. This enabled us to recognise that the resource could not only be used to work with young men but also to raise issues with young women.

Training and guidance

If your resource comes as part of a training pack, make sure that the training or guidance notes you develop are clear and simple to use. Remember that what might be clear to you may be totally confusing to someone else. You should also consider that users – youth workers, teachers or health education workers – will engage with young men in different settings and each of these settings will have an effect on the appropriateness of the resource. Your guidance notes may need to point this out.

Users

Your users may be male, female, parents, professional workers and/or young people themselves. Think about this when developing your resource. If it can only be used by male professional workers, for example, this will limit its circulation and its potential impact.

Conclusion

Developing resources is a time-consuming and often frustrating process. You will need to be committed to the issue and clear as to the purpose in order to generate the energy necessary to complete the fundraising and development. You will need to be brave and take risks. When developing your resource, follow your instincts and be prepared for criticism. Young men are very rarely seen as positive contributors to society and your effort may often be challenged as being a waste of time or creating extra work targeted at those who cause the most trouble. Remember: you will never please everyone or meet everyone's need.

Key issues for practitioners

- Working with young men can be hard, and tools which help communication are vital.
- Developing resources is time-consuming and can be frustrating. It requires workers to be clear about their purpose and committed in both the fundraising and development phases.

Practical pointers

- Think about your target audience and ensure they will be able to identify with any characters you create.
- Make sure the resource content is appropriate for the target group of men.
- Consider men's attitudes and feelings about the subject.
- Get a balance between realism and the health education issues so that they are reflected in appropriate settings and forms of communication.

8
Psychosexual therapy

Judi Keshet-Orr

This chapter covers:

- clients
- issues in therapy
- sex therapy
- the therapist's role
- key issues for practitioners
- practical pointers.

Introduction

As a woman working with men in a psychosexual and relationship setting for a number of years, I have found the environment both challenging and thought-provoking. Men present
with a variety of emotional and psychological issues, which
affect and inhibit their sexual lives and functioning. It is rarely
a simple physical cause of a sexual dysfunction that precipitates
the request for therapy. Many sexual difficulties are emotional
in origin; however, men who present with a physical difficulty,
for example with diabetes or multiple sclerosis, tend to have
some emotional issues to deal with which accompany their
physical condition. There is usually a parallel process and issues
can rarely be defined as purely physical or emotional. Physical
difficulties, particularly in the area of sexuality, are the ones
which men seem to have a great deal of difficulty in describing.
Men often see it as an affront to their masculinity to disclose
that they have difficulty ejaculating or sustaining an erection, or
that their penis is sore due to excessive or inappropriate masturbation. And men's sexual performance can be affected by
fear of pregnancy, infertility or subfertility.

A commonly held belief in the profession is that both men and women prefer talking to women. Quite how that impacts on male practitioners is a question which has only recently started to be addressed. It is, in my view, a dangerous and counterproductive assumption to make.

This chapter addresses psychosexual issues in the context of the couple relationship. Some of the ideas expounded here will also have significance for the therapist–client relationship.

Clients

In my own clinical settings in the NHS and in private practice, approximately 60% of the men who attend, either on their own or with their partners, are in heterosexual relationships. The remainder identify themselves as either gay or bisexual. The age range of men seeking sex therapy is extremely broad. In my NHS work the youngest man requesting therapy was 17 years old. He was a worker in the sex industry who had been referred by GU medicine for erectile failure. The oldest was a man of 73 who was bewildered and saddened at his loss, as he perceived it, of his sexual appetite and prowess. This man had been referred via his GP.

The age of men seeking help has changed since the mid-1990s: I now see an increasing number in the older age range asking for help. Perhaps a contributory factor is that men no longer believe that sex and their sexual needs will simply disappear or evaporate when they approach retirement age. Partners clearly play a role in this. Women and men are accepting that sex is not only for the young and/or for procreational purposes. Additionally there is much pleasure to be gained from the comfort and security of an established relationship in which sex and sensuality can play an important part. It is my belief that in general terms, those who have been part of the political changes since the 1980s have a greater sense of what they need, want and deserve.

As a sex therapist I will talk with my clients about the effects of ageing, and in some cases discuss the accommodation which will be required to incorporate these effects into their sexual relationship. In some instances even sex therapy with clients of over 65 has a psycho-educational input.

Although I see a higher proportion of heterosexual men and couples, it would be foolhardy to assume that heterosexual men have a higher degree of sexual difficulties. It is more probable that gay and bisexual men attend for therapy in the many gay affirmative and specialist agencies that are available. If I look at the ethnic and culturally diverse range of clients who attend for sex therapy in my private practice, the highest proportion of couples who attend are engaged in a transcultural relationship where the parties come from religiously and ethnically differing backgrounds. In the hospital clinic I oversee and coordinate, the largest proportion of the men attending are of Greek Cypriot origin, followed by Bangladeshis. This clearly reflects the ethnic composition of the area the hospital serves. Colleagues who work in other NHS settings report a different ethnic and cultural mix, largely dependent on the make-up of the local residents. Sadly the failure to attend for appointments is substantially higher in the NHS than in private practice. Whilst we could form some opinions about these differences in attendance rates, it is not within the scope of this chapter to do so.

Issues in therapy

The most common issues, in my experience, which men bring to therapy include:

- premature ejaculation
- erectile failure
- retarded ejaculation
- loss of desire
- sexual orientation confusion
- relationship issues, which generally focus on poor communication skills
- sex addiction
- the effects of ageing
- nonconsummation
- survivors of sexual abuse and incest
- penis size complex.

A particularly interesting area to work in is that of loss of desire or reduced sexual interest. As a presenting issue it often camouflages other problems, such as depression, alcohol or drug dependency, negative body image, fear of intimacy, or anxieties related to imposed or adopted morality. Many men will come up with a variety of attendant 'excuses' rather than confront the real or underlying issues.

This is also an interesting area to look at when we try to ascertain what exactly is 'normal' in terms of frequency of sexual activity. In a MORI/Esquire poll of 1992, the majority of men stated that they had sex two or three times a week. Only 2% stated that they had sex more than once a day. Anecdotal reports from men, by contrast, place the frequency of sexual activity more in line with the poll's 2% of respondents. I must question therefore the accuracy of such reports. Bradford (1995) claims that most men are 'natural exuberant risk takers ... sexually predatory ... [and] cursed by having to live up to society's macho image – 'real men don't cry'. Shame and embarrassment are feelings that traditionally have not been a recognised feature of men presenting in therapy. Much mythology abounds, particularly concerning the feelings and thought processes of men in therapy. It is only recently that men have been asked what they need and want from the therapeutic domain. Male-affirmative therapy and counselling are, at this stage, still subjects that exercise the minds and hearts of therapists and counsellors.

Sex therapy

Sex therapy in its modern form in the UK has its origins in the 1960s, and has come from a medical, behavioural and psychodynamic model. It is only since the mid-1990s that the influence of humanistic integrative therapy has made inroads into the work. Humanistic integrative therapy aims to be openly dialogie with both clients and peers and includes techniques from Gestalt, Transactional Analysis (TA) and Transpersonal therapy, amongst others. Practitioners attempt to include sociological and psychological research in their understanding. Many of you will no doubt be familiar with the traditional Masters and Johnson style of sex therapy which encourages clients to undertake many 'homework' tasks, and feed back to the counsellor or therapist on a weekly basis their success or failure. This method invites a parent/teacher/child interaction in the therapeutic domain, and leaves little scope for empowerment and self-direction. In my experience men can find this model difficult – it is often resonant of school and adult criticism and control. However, I do not wish to dismiss this methodology completely. It can, paradoxically, by its very nature be a powerful and useful tool in the therapeutic process, allowing more cautious men to work within a framework which is easily understandable and manageable.

This example is of a man who elected to have sex therapy and who previously had no experience of therapy or counselling. He presented with loss of passion – his description. A heterosexual man, who was in a long-term partner relationship and who had three young children, he led an active and stimulating working life where he was validated and appreciated for what he did. His sex life had for some considerable time been a source of disappointment to him. He felts undesired, lonely and perhaps most significantly, did not feel cherished. He was, however, committed to his relationship and family. This client had had these feelings for a number of years. His sex life was sporadic and it was always he who initiated sexual activity. His partner did not enjoy sexual activity but was supportive and tender in many other ways in the relationship. He masturbated regularly, using fantasy erotica.

This client had remained monogamous and had channelled his energies into developing his career and his role as a father and available parent to his children. He was disappointed with his relationship. He was confused that in his early 40s he found himself in a virtually celibate relationship. This did not fit in any way with the image he had hoped for himself, nor with the way in which he outwardly presented himself in the world.

He stated he was neither happy nor depressed; he was to some extent numb. I suggested that he had developed this numbness as a vehicle to protect himself against the pain of his absent sensual, emotional and sexual experience in his partner relationship. As a practitioner I needed to challenge some of his belief systems, act as advocate, invite change and act as a reflective therapist who could hold his sadness and disappointment. My task was neither to separate him from his relationship nor keep him in it, but to work with his desire to explore and resolve the issues that he had brought. Whilst this may not be the 'traditional' form of sex therapy I have no doubt that it falls within the remit of this work. This man's struggle with his sexual and sensual inner experience juxtaposed with his external experience informed the work. We looked at what he believed he deserved, what his rights were and how he might take responsibility for meeting his sexual and intimacy needs.

Other male clients have recounted their relief at having the opportunity to discuss intimate sexual matters in a safe and confidential environment. To be able to discuss their fears, anxieties and problems without fear of humiliation and ridicule is rare.

A client aged 45 who suffered from long-term erectile failure and premature ejaculation stated quite clearly that despite his initial embarrassment he was sorry that he had not taken the step to have therapy earlier in his life. This client was referred through GU medicine and had been offered injections to deal with his lack of erection. He had used the injection twice with his partner, and what they lacked in spontaneity they gained in a hard sustained erection for 3 hours. Having achieved this, they re-evaluated the potential for their long-term sex lives and chose to enter sex therapy. This man stated that he needed to go through the experience of self-injecting and all that this procedure evoked before he could allow himself the 'indulgence' of therapy.

Psychosexual and relationship work has for some time informed the arena of women's therapy; more recently I see it informing the world of men's therapy as well. Psychosexual therapy is a specialism; it differs in subtle ways from the more generalist approaches to counselling and therapy. Sexuality informs and impacts on most therapeutic relationships, but the specificity of this work and the mandate which sex therapists are offered by their clients is different. Clients in many differing areas of healthcare, social work and general practice environments present sexual difficulties. I would suggest that unless the practitioner, advisor or worker has had specialist training in this domain, there is potential for inappropriate advice, counselling or guidance to be given, which would result in the client being the poorer and the 'carer' feeling bewildered and confused.

A valuable resource for practitioners and clients alike is Zilbergeld's *The New Male Sexuality* (1999). This publication goes a long way in confronting some of the more damaging mythology around men's sexuality. A considerable amount of this mythology is brought into the consulting room. I would make a distinction between myth and fantasy. Fantasy is relatively widely used in sex therapy. Fantasies about positive outcomes, discussion about sexual fantasies which could be brought into the reality of the client's world – these are all part of what might take place within the therapy session. The use of imagery or guided fantasy may also form part of the therapeutic strategy. Myths, however, which hinder or distress the client, are to be explored and dispelled. A study by Baker & De Silva (1998) referred to nine myths which were relatively easy to confront. Daines explores the whole issue of sexual myths and their use or mis-use in an article in the *Journal of the Association of Sexual and Marital Therapists* (Daines 1990). This quarterly journal, since renamed *Sexual and Relationship Therapy*, is a valuable source of information for sex therapists, reflecting current trends and therapeutic changes in the field.

Humanistic integrative therapy combined with psychosexual therapy can be very powerful. Working with couples or individuals using these two models allows the therapist to focus the work and to use the couple's own awareness to facilitate change. The therapist needs to hold the boundaries and inform the clients, for whom working with 'what is' rather than 'what is not' is often confrontational and painful. We work with reality and what can be translated into reality. We also work with what must be left within the world of fantasy or unrealistic goals.

The therapist's role

As a sex therapist I will often have one of the most intimate relationships possible with a couple or individual without having sex. I will ask the client what they do, how they do it, where they do it, what they think, feel and desire. I will have to resist the 'tell us what to do' syndrome. It is often a strange experience for a man to have a mature woman with whom to share and discuss such intimate issues. The possible projection onto me as oracle, whore, mother or sexual fantasy object is clear, so professional supervision is of vital importance and ethically essential when performing this work.

Cultural and ethnic beliefs and attitudes also inform the work. As a therapist I need to be aware of the differences and similarities between my world and that of my clients. For example, it would be of little value for me to ask an orthodox Jewish man to spend some of his time developing masturbation techniques, self- and sensual-awareness exercises coupled with the viewing of sexually explicit educational video material. In many cases the therapy has to be adapted and changed to suit the client, not the other way round. The sex therapist needs to possess a high degree of flexibility, without losing sight of the mandate which the client has offered for the work.

An attempt to describe fully a sexual difficulty appropriate to therapy can be difficult. Inevitably there are subtleties which may be related to age, ethnicity, health status, sexual orientation and preference, and secondary or intermittent difficulties. The definition of what is normal or abnormal, healthy or unhealthy is often subjective – what may be beyond the bounds of acceptability to me may fall within the bounds of acceptable behaviour for the client, and vice versa. It is unrealistic to think that I can work with all clients and they can all work with me. It is also unrealistic to think that sex therapy will facilitate change for all clients, so an initial assessment session for both client and therapist is vital.

Conclusion

Sex therapy from an integrative perspective is a fascinating and challenging area of work. It is not simply a method or a range of techniques. It is, at its best, a creative and profound way of working, where the meaning for the client forms the foundation of the therapy; where there is an acceptance that without pain and change there can be no growth; where there will be a level of self-disclosure which allows the client to reorganise cognitively and somatically in order to achieve his stated goals. It is by its very nature an interactive and sensitive environment for both client and therapist.

References

Baker C D, De Silva P 1998 The relationship between male sexual dysfunction and belief in Zilbergeld's Myths: an empirical investigation. Journal for Sexual and Marital Therapy 3:229–238

Bradford N 1995 Men's health matters: the complete A–Z of male health. Vermillion, London

Daines B 1990 Sexual myths and sex therapists. Journal of the Association of Sexual and Marital Therapists 5(2):149–154

Zilbergeld B 1999 The new male sexuality. Bantam, London

Key issues for practitioners

■ Men come to psychosexual therapy with a variety of issues both physical and emotional e.g. premature ejaculation, loss of desire, relationship issues, penis size.

■ It is only recently that men have been asked what they want and need from therapists and counsellors and so male-positive work is still developing.

■ Sex therapy has come traditionally from a medical model e.g. the Masters and Johnson approach. Only recently has it begun to include more humanistic approaches. Some men have found the traditional model difficult.

Practical pointers

■ The therapist can usefully challenge belief systems about sex and relationships.

■ The task of the therapist is not to separate or keep together a couple but to work with the client's desire to explore and resolve his own issues.

■ Men may present sexual difficulties in different areas of healthcare, such as general practice or social work. Unless the professional has had specialist training there is the danger that inappropriate counselling or advice will be given.

■ Professional supervision for therapists is very important.

9

The new men's media

Peter Baker

This chapter covers:

- who's spending the pennies?
- does it add up?
- getting stuck in
- how to do it
- the upshot
- key issues for practitioners
- practical pointers.

Introduction

The glossy, middle-shelf, consumer magazines for men are an astonishing publishing phenomenon. When *Arena* was launched in 1986, followed by *GQ* in 1988, many doubted whether men would buy them. By early 2000, there were 10 major titles with total sales exceeding 1.5 million copies a month. Health issues feature prominently in many of them – in fact, they have become as much a fixture as football, Ferraris and front-cover pin-ups.

These magazines offer one of the few significant sources of health information for men. A typical doctor's waiting room is unlikely to have leaflets or posters on erectile dysfunction, male infertility or testicular cancer, but if there are copies of *Men's Health*, *FHM* or *Men's Fitness* in the magazine rack, then a man will almost certainly find articles on these important topics. Even though obesity, lack of physical activity and poor diet are major causes of ill health in men, the men's magazines contain just about the only source of easily accessible information targeted specifically at them on how to lead a healthier lifestyle.

An analysis of one month's magazines shows the breadth of health issues covered. In February 2000, *Men's Health* (monthly sales 218 724 according to ABC, the Audit Bureau of Circulation) included articles on stress management, sexual problems and the health benefits of walking. *Men's Fitness* (no ABC figure) focused on weight control, *FHM Bionic* (no ABC figure) on complementary medicine and tackling addictions, and *Maxim* (monthly sales 310 096) on healthy eating. Meanwhile *FHM* (monthly sales 701 500) devoted seven pages to answering readers' questions about a wide range of physical and mental health problems, including coping with bereavement, premature ejaculation and shaving rashes.

In the last few years, the emergence of several specialist men's health and fitness titles has meant that a few magazines have significantly reduced their health coverage. *Esquire* (monthly sales 100 380), *GQ* (145 144) and *Arena* (46 777) for instance now include very little on health, although *GQ* does publish a substantial quarterly health and fitness supplement called *GQ Active*. *Later* (no ABC figure) provides just two health pages, comprising several 'shorts' on a variety of topics (in February 2000 these included antioxidants, the health benefits of prayer, and Pilates, a method of body-conditioning). The most 'laddish' of the middle-shelf men's magazines, *Loaded* (384 351), has consistently provided no health information for its readers.

A survey of the health coverage in the first 18 issues of *Maxim* (May 1995 – October 1996) shows that it addressed almost all of what were then the *Health of the Nation* key target areas (there were articles on coronary heart disease and stroke, cancer, mental illness and sexual health) along with back pain, eye problems, oral health and gastrointestinal disorders. All the magazines which cover health consistently pay more attention to prevention rather than treatments and there tend to be few sensationalised stories about rare and frightening conditions. There is a surprising openness to complementary medicine and, although some health professionals might take issue with the emphasis placed on certain conditions, there appear to be few factual errors.

Who's spending the pennies?

Although a significant number of men are buying one or more of the magazines covering health, they are drawn from a relatively narrow group. Each publication has its particular market niche, but the majority of the readers of all of them are between about 20 and 40, white-collar (usually professional) and heterosexual. (Only *Attitude*, which sells 55 000 copies a month according to the publisher's own figures, is gay-oriented, although by no means gay-exclusive.) Three-quarters of those buying *Men's Health*, and two-thirds of *Maxim* readers, are in social classes ABC1; the average *Maxim* reader is aged 27 and enjoys an annual post-tax income of £17,600.

Esquire defines its 'core buyer' as being 'in the pre-family lifestage, likely to be between 25–30 with commitments to his job, partner and home. Well-educated, career-minded and successful, he has reached a stage in his life when he is confident about who he is, what he wants and where he is going'. Given the almost complete absence of coverage of black and ethnic minority men and their issues, it can reasonably be assumed that the editors of all the magazines assume that most of their readers are white.

While the magazines' readers are clearly not the men in worst health, this does not mean they do not have legitimate health needs. Younger men are particularly at risk of testicular cancer and can benefit from information about self-examination. This age group is also likely to be more concerned than many older men about issues relating to fertility and sexually transmitted diseases. And although relatively few men under 40 are affected by heart disease, they could still reduce their future risk if they followed the magazines' advice to adopt a healthier lifestyle by eating better, exercising more, stopping smoking and reducing stress. It is also possible that, simply by covering health, the magazines are helping to normalise and legitimise the notion that it is acceptable for any man to be concerned about his physical and emotional wellbeing.

Does it add up?

A more profound criticism of the magazines' health coverage is that it tends to be sandwiched between a much larger number of other articles that appear to encourage distinctly unhealthy activities. Most of the magazines devote considerable attention to high-risk sports (e.g. mountaineering, motor car racing, bungee jumping) and to drinking alcohol. The sexual explicitness with which women are commonly portrayed does little to encourage an awareness of the importance of negotiating and practising safer sex. There are very few articles which seek to explore the nature of masculinity itself or encourage a 'softer' maleness, both of which might help men feel more comfortable about paying greater attention to their health.

The magazines also tend to present health to their readers in the context of personal appearance or achievement. In other words, much of the health advice is not actually about being healthy for its own sake; rather, it is about how to look good or how to succeed at work or with women. When any of the magazines emphasise, for instance, the importance of regular aerobic exercise and low-fat foods, it is rarely with the intention of helping their readers avoid heart disease; the principal aim is to help them achieve a flat, muscular stomach. There is also the distinct possibility that the magazines' relentless emphasis on aspirational self-improvement may contribute towards a self-consciousness, if not insecurity, that will not do much to improve men's mental health.

Despite these problems, the magazines may well have stumbled on an effective way of getting health messages across to younger men, a group usually considered very difficult to reach. It may not be particularly palatable to many, but large numbers of such men are interested in cars, football and the sex lives of female film stars. If that package also contains some useful information that reduces the harm men do to themselves, or even improves their health, then the magazines may be providing something more significant than mere entertainment.

The magazines' avoidance of 'worthy' public health messages and their focus on men's everyday and immediate concerns is an important part of their approach. Telling men to stop smoking because they might get lung cancer in 30 years is probably less likely to have an impact on behaviour than pointing out that they could expect firmer and longer-lasting erections within a few months. Similarly, suggesting men eat less fat and more carbohydrate is more likely to be taken seriously if presented as a means of improving their sports performance in the short term, rather than a way of avoiding heart disease in the long. The magazines' frequent use of humour, particularly a form of self-deprecating irony, is also a central part of their health coverage. Making health funny may well have the function of disarming the belief of many readers that it is not really their issue.

Getting stuck in

So long as these magazines remain one of the few means of reaching large numbers of men with health messages – and while men's health remains so poor – it makes sense for those with a commitment to improving men's health to seek to work with them to maintain, expand and (hopefully) improve their health coverage. But health professionals have not yet shown much enthusiasm for either influencing the content of articles or placing advertisements. In part, this is because some health promoters do not yet accept the case for gender-specific targeting. They would argue, for instance, that a single health message on, say, skin cancer is equally applicable to men and women even though it is now clear that each gender has a very different attitude to sun-tanning and using skin care products. Other health workers, meanwhile, do not believe that men's magazines are an appropriate vehicle for transmitting health messages to men. They might argue that it makes more sense to work with magazines dedicated to sport, cars or hobbies like angling, because they tend to have much broader male audiences than the lifestyle publications. But those types of magazine do not regularly cover health issues, so it would be much harder to generate coverage in them. In any event, of course, working with one type of publication does not preclude working with any other.

However, the lack of contact between health professionals and men's magazines is not just the responsibility of the former. Some of the journalists writing about men's health are not primarily health writers and therefore do not see it as a priority to develop long-term relationships with health workers. Moreover, because much of the health information in the magazines is presented in relatively short articles, it is often compiled from medical reference books, journals and press cuttings, further reducing the opportunities for personal contact between journalists and experts. But all journalists and magazines are (or should be) constantly looking for new and interesting stories and will usually respond to good ideas, wherever they come from.

How to do it

So how can health professionals begin to work more effectively with the men's magazines? The starting points must be:

- an acceptance of the importance of tackling men's health problems
- an acknowledgement of the necessity for gender-specific health messages
- a recognition that the men's magazines provide a means of reaching a significant and growing constituency of men.

For those who might be deterred by disapproval of much of the content of most men's magazines (including the celebration of 'traditional' masculinity and the proliferation of sexist images of women), it is worth considering whether the potential for harm reduction is sufficient to make working with the magazines acceptable. For those who are deterred by disapproval of the press generally, it is worth reflecting on which other media can facilitate communication with important target groups so quickly or cheaply.

It is vital to read the magazines to understand their approach and to get a sense of what issues they are likely – and not likely – to want to cover. Given their readership profile, it is highly unlikely they would be interested in covering new treatments for Alzheimer's disease or the importance of cervical screening, whereas articles on, say, condoms, stress, sexual problems or sports injuries are much more likely to be published.

Health practitioners must exercise their creativity and work out how to fit their agenda into that of the magazines. For instance, a campaign to encourage sensible drinking could be worked into an article on how to avoid developing a beer gut; an initiative to get men to seek help for depression could be related to an article on splitting up with a partner. Most health organisations will have a press/publicity officer who should be able to advise about how best to present information to a range of different publications.

Regional or local health organisations should remember that they stand as much chance of obtaining coverage for their campaigns as better-known national agencies. For example, a local initiative promoting testicular self-examination could well generate an article if it went beyond the traditional advice and was linked, say, to case studies of men who had been successfully treated for cancer.

It is important to understand the publishing timescale of a monthly magazine. The July issue of a magazine will normally be published in early June. The text will probably be with the printers by early May and the copy deadline for writers could be mid-April. Articles could well be commissioned up to 4–8 weeks before that date. This means that for an article on preventing skin cancer to appear in the July issue, the magazine should be contacted no later than mid-March, over 14 weeks before the date on the magazine's cover. These long publication schedules continually cause problems for everyone involved in magazine publishing. The answer for those seeking to influence the editorial content is either to be very well organised or to push for coverage of stories which are not linked to a particular time of year.

It is useful to find out the name of the health editor (normally this is printed among the list of contributors towards the front of the magazine) so that information and ideas can be sent directly to him or her. Health editors work in different ways. Some prefer to have ideas sent to them by post or fax, while others respond better to a telephone call. Generally, until a particular editor's preference is known, it is better to post material in the first instance and to follow this up with a phone call a week later if no reply has been received. The lack of an immediate response does not necessarily mean that the idea is a bad one; rather, it is likely to reflect the fact that the editor is busy meeting deadlines and sifting through many other unsolicited ideas and suggestions from public relations companies, health organisations and freelance journalists who are looking for work. Many of the health editors are in fact freelance journalists themselves and it can also take time for post or telephone messages to be forwarded to their own place of work.

Even if suggestions appear to be disappearing into a vacuum, it is always worth persisting. If the health editor regularly receives information from an agency, he or she may well remember it as a potentially good source of expertise. This means that the organisation could well end up being contacted – and quoted – by a journalist pursuing a story (which may, or may not, be directly related to any ideas you have submitted).

The upshot

Like them or loathe them, men's magazines are here to stay. The biggest-selling title, *FHM*, now boasts a larger circulation than

Cosmopolitan. A new title is now launched almost every year. With the majority covering health issues, there is clearly an opportunity for health professionals to influence their content. At a time when the Government hopes to raise the profile of men's health, when new men's health charities and campaigns are being launched and when more health authorities are beginning to recognise the importance of tackling men's health problems, the magazines offer a ready-made vehicle for creative and well-targeted initiatives. Although getting coverage in men's magazines is just one of many ways of improving men's health, there is little doubt that it could play a significant part in eliminating one of the biggest, and most intractable, of all the health inequalities.

Key issues for practitioners

- Men's magazines offer one of the few accessible sources of information for men about health issues.
- These magazines pay significantly more attention to prevention than to treatment.
- Articles don't usually question assumptions about masculinity and health, and often present issues in the context of personal appearance or achievement.

Practical pointers

- Men's magazines are a useful channel for getting health messages to a younger group of men usually considered by practitioners as being hard to reach.
- Health practitioners should try to work with these magazines, and make the most of the opportunities they offer.
- To do this effectively, health professionals need to get to know the magazines and understand how they work, both in terms of style and more practically in terms of production timescales.
- Making contact with the health editor of a particular magazine and being persistent are important.
- Regional organisations have as much chance as national ones of getting coverage of an issue, provided it is tackled creatively.

10

Self-help groups

Phil Williams

Introduction

WCT Phoneline For Men with Cancer (formerly Mind Over Matter) is a self-help group for men who are concerned about, or who have been diagnosed with, testicular cancer (TC). We talked to Phil Williams, a founder member.

How did the group get started?

The trigger was the death of a young man from testicular cancer. His mother felt so angry that not enough was known about it that she lobbied the consultant who had been involved in her son's case to do something to help provide support and increase awareness of TC. Very often self-help groups like ours are formed when someone either dies or is affected by a potentially fatal illness.

In our case the consultant wrote to a large number of his patients inviting them and their families to an open meeting, where he proposed setting up local support groups made up of ex-patients. By the end of the meeting a small number of men had agreed to form four local groups and with a lot of support, help and encouragement from the consultant and our regional cancer charity, the Wessex Cancer Trust (WCT), the groups were started. We are fortunate to be supported by and linked with the Wessex Cancer Trust, an independent charity that tackles the problems of cancer in Dorset, Hampshire, Wiltshire, the Isle of Wight and the Channel Islands. The Trust supports many aspects of cancer care and aims to help people understand more about the disease. It works towards cancer prevention wherever possible and provides facilities for early detection and screening.

We named the group Mind Over Matter because we felt cancer is also a psychological battle for many of us, and we have to cope mentally with the different thoughts, feelings and emotions we experience.

What were the main issues at the beginning for the individual men and for the group?

Initially we had a problem about getting someone to take on organising the group. We were all men who had jobs, so it was very difficult. None of us had any experience of starting or running a self-help support group. An illustration of this problem was that within 12 months of the four groups starting, only one was still in existence. In those critical early days and weeks, without the support of the consultant, the WCT and some dedicated professionals we would probably not have carried on. Our learning curve was steep and just deciding the best place to meet was fraught with difficulty. With an issue like TC you have to draw members from quite a wide geographical area. We tried the hospital, church halls, public houses, hotel lounges and offices. The remaining group, which is based in Southampton, has met in all these places. For some members the hospital brought back unpleasant memories of their treatment, others found the church hall too formal, the public house worked quite well for established members but not for new ones and the hotel lounge was too public.

For us as individuals initially the issue was about normalising our experience, talking about it with others who shared the experience for the first time. But I suppose we learned how to run it by default really. The difficulty is that men do not naturally gravitate to support groups, especially to discuss their feelings with strangers. It can be a daunting prospect to join any group of strangers, even for purely social reasons.

Did you have a clear set of aims from the outset?

With the help of the WCT we decided on the main aims of the group. These were to:

- provide support through befriending
- increase awareness of TC and promote self-examination
- fundraise locally for the WCT.

Why didn't the group recruit new members?

We're not sure why. We thought our close link with the local hospital and the consultant would provide us with a number of new members. This, sadly, has not been the case. Even though the leaflets produced for us by the WCT are distributed to new and existing TC patients, the number of enquiries we have received in 8 years has been just two, and yet we are told that between 50 and 70 new patients are diagnosed each year in our area. I suspect the group wasn't properly advertised by the hospital. I suppose they were just very busy people, but I'm not really sure why recruitment was so hard.

Does the group still function as a support group or has it more of a lobbying, advocacy type of role now?

Mostly it's an advocacy group now. We do support each other but most of what we do is about informing and supporting others outside of the group. We still need to do more work to determine how a service like ours can be delivered to, or accessed by, these men at the right time and in the right way. We believe the starting point is to clearly state what the type and level of our service is and how we intend to deliver it.

We provide the opportunity for men and their families who are affected by the diagnosis of TC to talk to someone who has been through the same or a similar experience. Our service is confidential. This means we do not keep personal details, only the number of enquiries received, and we do not offer medical advice. We are fortunate in having the additional backup of training sponsored by the WCT to ensure that we provide a quality service to those who seek our help. The WCT also offers support and professional counselling for any of our members who become emotionally affected through trying to help others.

Other than the telephone phoneline you run for men and their partners, what else do you do?

The WCT keep us supplied with leaflets to help increase awareness of TC. Last year we received lots of requests for information from health professionals. Gradually over the last 8 years more and more organisations have contacted us to ask if they can register our group on their database and sometimes on their internet website. Over the years we have contacted other national charities to ask if they would include us in their literature. This networking with other organisations has worked well for us and we now receive enquiries from throughout the UK, about 80% of which are from health professionals and 20% from concerned men or their partners. We try to increase awareness of TC through:

- sending out leaflets
- appearing on local radio and television
- articles in local papers
- talks in schools and companies
- linking with health professionals.

What do you feel has been your main achievement over the years?

I suppose the main thing is that those men who are failing to go to their doctor we encourage to get checked out. The message we give them is that it's right and responsible to be concerned about your health. Also, we've been able to sympathise with their experience. They know we've been through it too.

If you were to offer advice to anyone setting up a self-help group on a men's health issue what would it be?

Approach it like a business. You need to research the market and see what men need around that particular issue. If I was starting again I would like to have the time to do that. The important issues to ask yourself are:

- Why are you starting this group?
- What are your objectives?
- How are you going to finance the group?
- Where are you going to meet?
- How are you going to get men to attend?
- How are you going to run the group meetings?
- What level of support can you provide?
- What (emotional) protection have you for yourself and your members?
- What are the ground rules for your group?
- How will you promote your group's activities?
- How are you going to interface with health professionals?
- Is there anyone else who is already providing this service (or another group or organisation you can link in with)?
- What are your long-term objectives?

This list is not exhaustive, but we believe that unless you are clear about why you are starting a group and how it will operate, like so many businesses, it will fail. The national charity Cancerlink provide a *Starting a Support Group* information pack as well as *Good Practice Guidelines* for cancer self-help groups, and training.

The other major thing is to try and capture men's attention at a time when they are likely to be receptive – in a GP setting for example. This is where most men start to discover something might be wrong.

What is the way ahead for work on testicular cancer?

I think that awareness is what's important. The success rate for treatment is very good. It's a young man's disease so I'd like to see information targeted at younger men in the education system. That's probably the single most important thing we could do.

For the future we see a growing need for collaboration and a bringing together of the multiplicity of information and support services available. There is undoubtedly duplication of both effort and information that in today's modern cost-led environment is unacceptable, especially when these funds are becoming ever more difficult to raise in the voluntary sector.

Key issues for practitioners

■ Men do not naturally join support groups, especially to discuss feelings with strangers. It is important to capture men's attention when they might be receptive e.g. in a primary care setting.

■ More work is needed to determine how self-help groups can be delivered and accessed by men at the right time and in the right way.

■ You should be clear about why you are starting a self-help group and how it will operate.

■ There is a need for collaboration with health care professionals and other self-help groups, and the wide range of available information needs to be rationalised.

Practical pointers

■ Approach setting up a self-help group as you would a business.

■ Ask lots of tough questions about finance, location, objectives, ground rules and promotion.

■ Get advice from those with experience in running a support group.

11

A community health approach to men's health

David Hart and Tony Mays

> **This chapter covers:**
>
> ■ context
> ■ the project
> ■ evaluation
> ■ challenges
> ■ benefits
> ■ follow-up ventures
> ■ setting up a project
> ■ the way ahead
> ■ key issues for practitioners
> ■ practical pointers.

Introduction

This chapter presents an evaluation of three 12-week Good Health for Men Groups (a total of 36 sessions) run between October 1994 and December 1995. The project was run jointly by a community mental health nurse working for Community Health Sheffield Trust and a social worker from Sheffield Family and Community Services. Funding initially came from Sheffield Health and Community Health Sheffield.

Context

We felt that we needed to look at issues around 'body, mind and spirit', as they seemed to us to be intrinsically linked. Men often do not want to take responsibility for their own health and wellbeing, or if they do, they do not know how to go about accessing relevant services.

We had begun working together in a mental health setting, but in 1993 we began to look at ways of addressing men's health issues from a wider perspective. In addition to our own observations and experience, various policy initiatives on a local, regional and national level indicated that there was a need for preventative and health promotional work with men. These included:

- The *Health of the nation* key area of mental health and the primary target of reduction in suicide rates (Department of Health 1992).

- The objectives of the Community Health Sheffield and Local Authority Mental Health Strategy.

- East Midlands Men's Health Network's initiatives around men's health.

- Our increasing awareness of the stresses in men's lives and how their experiences and expectations impinge on their physical and psychological wellbeing.

- The Chief Medical Officer's Report (Calman 1993) high-lighting men's health as an area in need of greater attention.

- A further report by Rod Griffiths, the Regional Director of Public Health for the West Midland Authority (Griffiths 1994) illustrating the gender gap in health and how health was related to poverty (e.g. male mortality rates are lower in more affluent areas).

- Media interest in men and health had grown (e.g. there was coverage of gender-specific illnesses such as prostate and testicular cancer).

Over the years our experience gained through running health-focused men's groups had led us to the view that there were many common experiences, patterns of behaviour and areas of concern which our group members shared not only with each other but also with men more generally. In addition, the separation of psychological issues from physical and social/environment factors seemed to us to be artificial and restrictive. Consequently we developed ideas for a health promotional approach to men's health, which incorporated education, discussions and personal development within a group work setting. Our aim was to provide the opportunity for men to meet together to extend their knowledge about their own health and to discuss health concerns in a 'safe' setting.

The project

The project was initially funded for a year by Sheffield Health and Community Health Sheffield. It was designed to look at physical, social and emotional health issues for men, who are often reluctant to acknowledge ignorance in these areas and unwilling to seek help with difficulties they might experience. It took the form of a 'rolling programme' of talks and discussions followed by a support group. Three cycles were envisaged, each lasting 12 weeks.

An open referral system was put into operation so that in principle any man in Sheffield could attend for all, some or one of the sessions. Information about the group appeared in the local press. Referrals in the main came from GPs, medical staff and colleagues in the mental health field.

Each 12-week course began with an introductory session in which every man could get a 'taste' of what was to come and to see if it was to his liking. In addition, if it was felt either by the referrer or the potential member himself that a pre-group individual appointment or telephone call would be helpful, then this was arranged. We attracted a wide range of men from as young as 20 to past retirement. Backgrounds varied from unemployed and disabled men to 'middle class' professionals.

Following the introductory meeting six sessions were arranged, run largely by outside specialists covering topics such as:

- depression and self harm
- body and soul
- media images of men
- drug and alcohol abuse
- stress at work
- looking after your kit and other bits.

Professional input ranged from physiotherapists and health visitors to workers in the voluntary sector who look after people with long-term mental health problems. In the last course we had a local GP and a pharmacist attending. These sessions were followed by five closed group sessions, in which group members were able to discuss in depth real issues surrounding the topics covered.

The original programme was the product of our views of the health needs of men, but the following two 12-week courses were significantly influenced by group members. The second group established strong mutual bonds and a common purpose which provided many ideas that were developed subsequently. For example, in the third group the idea had evolved of directly following up a specialist session with a discussion group on the subjects covered the previous week.

When the second course finished after 12 weeks, the participants formed themselves into a self-help group which was supported initially by Community Health Sheffield and now by Sheffield Healthline. By the time we did the third course we had devised individual action plans. They became an integral part of the process. Each member was asked to identify a health difficulty e.g. lack of confidence or depression, then, relating to what they had been doing in previous sessions, they put down their aim or plan to reduce their difficulty, along with a review date. In this way the members began to take responsibility for their own health.

Evaluation

At the beginning of each programme group members were asked to fill in a men's health questionnaire. The main concerns these revealed were:

- stress
- anxiety
- self-confidence.

Often these problems were related to other issues such as unemployment and loss.

Group evaluation forms were used at the end of the course and proved to be a valuable tool in examining the appropriateness and effectiveness of the project. The question 'Choose the most significant event during the course as a whole' elicited such responses as:

- 'I realised redundancy had a bigger effect on me than the deaths of two close old relatives.'

- 'I was able to tell something very traumatic, all the group listened. This was important to me because I had never been able to explain the effects this incident had on me before.'

Overall the main themes which emerged from these evaluations were:

- Input from and discussion with specialists was helpful.

- Increased confidence was gained through sharing experiences and learning that problems were not unique.

- Communication and support were key elements.

- More emphasis on physical health issues and on stress-related problems was requested.

Individual action plans were intended to focus the minds of group members on change and personal responsibility for their own health, as a consolidation of the information gained, experience shared and confidence exchanged during the course. We had a follow-up review after 3 months to look at the effectiveness of the course and the participants' action plans. The main themes to emerge were:

- Maintaining the impetus and motivation for change on one's own is difficult.

- Support is a key element.

- Benefits had come from increased knowledge, including the possibility of making more informed choices and having greater self-confidence

Other evaluation outcomes, including feedback from specialist facilitators, helped us to plan and structure subsequent courses. Generally the response of the 'specialists' was surprise at the immediate interest and enthusiasm the men showed in the subject areas. Discussion was always thoughtful and wide-ranging and seemed to belie the conventional wisdom that men are inarticulate about personal and emotional matters.

Weekly meetings and consultation with a colleague was essential in helping us maintain our own focus and also the momentum within the group. Our meetings served many purposes, from discussing practical matters to looking at individual styles and contributions within the group. We constantly refined and adjusted our approach through the meetings and examined our objectives. This was fed back to the group the following week. Much of our current thinking is the result of the interaction of our own deliberations with the views of group members.

An educational and training programme was developed in addition to the group sessions. This included a visual display plus leaflets and literature, talks and discussion groups, workshops and seminars, and local newspaper and radio publicity designed to raise the profile of men's health issues in Sheffield.

Challenges

Finding the right venue for the courses was problematic. It had to feel 'safe', as well as being conveniently located. It needed to be no more than one bus ride away, otherwise some of the men would have been deterred from attending the group.

One consequence of our professional backgrounds (in mental health) was that there tended to be a weighting towards men with mental health histories, as many of the referrals came via our colleagues who were aware of our project through internal publicity and word-of-mouth.

We advertised the courses as being open groups which men could 'dip into' as they wished. On reflection (and in fact this largely happened in practice) forming a closed group after a couple of sessions would seem to be preferable, as the members valued the developing trust and mutual support which the group afforded. Individuals joining mid-course were welcomed, but found it difficult to find a 'place' within the group.

Often the group offered the only opportunity men felt they had to talk, and for some the 12 weeks were not long enough. We feel there is a case for running a longer-term, more 'therapeutic' group, for men to move on to if they wish, as well as the other option of a self-help group.

Finding funding and appropriate accommodation for a self-help group was something of a problem. Once the facilitators withdrew from active involvement, other budgetary sources had to be sought.

Benefits

The benefits of the Good Health for Men Groups were as follows:

- The project gave men in Sheffield the opportunity of attending an educational, awareness-raising group focusing on the social, psychological and physical aspects of health for men.

- Discussion and the exchange of ideas and experiences enabled the men to look at their difficulties in a wider context.

- The groups developed a system of mutual support, giving the men the sense of being able to help others, rather than just being the recipients of help.

- The project helped significantly to change the attitudes and behaviour of participants. An example of this was increased confidence in seeking out and activating services and resources. Men became better informed and were more likely to seek help and advice on health issues than before attending the group.

- Lessons learned during the course led to some men taking more active steps to improve their health.

- The men developed skills and confidence in talking to each other and gained strength from a shared acknowledgement of their experiences.

- A self-help support group was established and remained active for 1 year following the end of our involvement.

Follow-up ventures

Since the project was completed at the end of 1996 we have continued to disseminate knowledge and information gained about men's health issues to other health and social service professionals.

We are separately working on a number of other projects relating to men's health and may restart the Good Health for Men Group at a later date. We have jointly set up the Sheffield Men's Health Forum, which brings together organisations working in men's health in the city to exchange ideas and information. One of us is at present involved in running a city-wide Male Violence Group for men who acknowledge their violent behaviour and want to change. It also offers support to their partners.

Community Health Sheffield has acknowledged the need to raise awareness in the city, and established a Men's Health Task Group, which we are both members of, to look at providing more relevant and accessible services for men.

Setting up a project

The therapeutic value and the cost-effectiveness of looking at men's health issues in a group rather than on an individual basis is beginning to be realised: men can be helped to be supportive and open with each other. We are often asked how we got started and how we managed to retain the men's interest. Our reply is: 'through reflection and experience'. We would advise anybody who wants to initiate and to develop work around men's health to look at the local perception of health needs in their community. Does your perception match the local health and community thinking on men's health? Make the most of people's skills by empowering them in the process of change within the group. Aims and objectives could centre around examining men's beliefs and behaviour. Encourage other disciplines inside and outside nursing to take part in the programme, to get a wider perspective on men's issues.

Be high profile about the group and use the local media to promote men's health in a positive way. Set up systems that can evaluate group outcomes in line with the rationale of the group, but keep them as simple as possible. Seek managerial support for your idea. Also, look for common interests that men can connect with. For example, we identified a way of interesting men by publicising what the programme would contain. This information was circulated not just amongst our health colleagues but at public amenities, libraries, sports centres – anywhere where men might meet.

Our success was due to looking at men's needs primarily, but not exclusively, through health. This model has been seen to be successful, in that colleagues have set up subsequent groups from a similar starting point. Once in the groups men readily look at other topics e.g. confidence building, personal awareness, sexuality – but if the group had been set up specifically to look at confidence building, for example, then hardly anyone would have turned up. Many men are still hanging on to the 'macho' image of control.

Our group showed that men are good at talking once they can identify difficulties with each other. Try to empower the men in the group. We did this by sharing the learning experiences not just of the men but of the facilitators as well. We adopted an open, honest stance in the group. Trust was quickly built up by varying the topics, seeking the participants' views, being flexible in approach, changing the programme in response to the group's needs. It is essential that you build in time for the group to reflect on issues that had been previously discussed. Ensure that you have sufficient time to run the group. This sounds obvious, but it is surprising how many people find that they have clashes with other commitments.

The way ahead

Men's health in the 21st century needs to be explored on several different levels. Two key areas of concern are:

1. research
2. central Government policy making.

We need to research ways of promoting men's health. Financial commitment from NHS trusts for yearly budgets to support the research is needed to find out, for example, how to interest men in addressing health issues. What models are most successful – group or individual work? How do we best get action around men's health into service provision?

Local initiatives such as ours can only take us so far towards addressing men's health needs. What we would like to see is some leadership from central Government to create a national framework (Men's Health Forum 1997). If this were in place, then perhaps local NHS trusts would release funding more readily. In particular, we need to take action urgently by providing services for young men while they are still at school, giving them the opportunity to examine the male role in today's society. Unless we tackle men's health from a national perspective, then suicide rates for young men may well continue to rise.

Key issues for practitioners

■ Men's confidence was increased by participating in small groups, specifically through sharing experiences and learning that their health problems were not unique.

■ The men gained a sense of helping others as well as being recipients of help.

■ It is difficult for men to maintain the changes made in the group if they lack ongoing support.

■ Participation in the programme increased men's confidence to seek out services and resources.

Practical pointers

■ Check out your perceptions of need within the local community with others.

■ Encourage a multidisciplinary approach.

■ Set up simple evaluation systems for the group.

■ Be flexible about the programme.

References

Calman K 1993 On the state of the public health – 1992. HMSO, London
Department of Health 1992 The health of the nation. HMSO, London
Griffiths R 1994 Agenda for Health. NHS Executive, West Midlands
Men's Health Forum 1997 Men's health audit report. Men's Health Forum

12

Promoting weight loss in men aged 40–55: the *Keeping It Up* campaign

David Wilkins

This chapter covers:

- focus groups
- campaign design
- objectives of the campaign
- introduction to evaluation
- involvement of workplaces
- level of participation
- administration
- physical outcomes for individual participants
- attitudinal changes in participants
- longer-term influence of participation
- key issues for practitioners
- practical pointers.

Introduction

Health promotion campaigns which aim to prevent coronary heart disease (CHD) in older men are notoriously difficult to design and sustain. This target group is widely held to be suspicious of health messages which carry with them the suggestion of a change in personal habits. For many people, indeed, the phrases 'middle-aged man' and 'set in his ways' are virtually synonymous! In fairness though, most people would recognise that the years of most concentrated family and work commitments are not those in which it is easy to find time and space to think about one's health. It is not only health professionals, however, who are aware that once men reach their 40s, their level of physical activity reduces, their weight increases and their risk of developing CHD greatly increases.

The central feature of the *Keeping It Up* campaign is an inter-workplace competition held over a 6-month period. Each workplace is represented by a team of six men. Team membership is limited to men aged 40–55 with a body mass index (BMI) of between 27 and 30. Points are awarded for reductions in the percentage body fat of individual team members. A monthly league table shows the relative points total of each team and a trophy is awarded at the end of the period to the 'league champions'. All participants receive a fitness screening at the beginning and end of the competition period and are offered education, support and encouragement to enable them to become more physically active and to eat more healthily.

The campaign, which is an initiative of HealthWorks, Dorset's Health Promotion Agency, has been run three times, the first time being from July to December 1995. Unless otherwise stated, references throughout this chapter are to the earlier of the two initiatives, which was formally evaluated.

Focus groups

The *Keeping It Up* campaign began with the premise that if we are to influence men in their 40s and 50s to look after their bodies, then we must first find out what is going on in their minds. Accordingly, we held a series of focus groups with men from a range of social and occupational backgrounds. It was in this process of creative consultation that the seeds of the campaign's subsequent success were sown.

From the focus groups we learned that:

- Men tend to rationalise away the health risks of an inactive lifestyle (e.g. it is 'natural' to be a bit overweight as one gets older – this does not mean that one is not 'fit').

- Whilst men may worry about losing their physical attractiveness, they consider a preoccupation with appearance to be a 'women's thing'.

- Men know little about the nutritional content of the food they eat.

- Some men regard 'exercise' as boring and time-consuming – others regard 'keeping fit' as 'middle class' and therefore not for them.

- On the whole, men prefer team sports to exercising alone.

- They like the element of competition in sport.

- They would be most interested in a health-promoting initiative if it took place in the workplace.

- Those who are less fit are awkward about exercising in the company of younger men who are in better shape.

Overall, participants in the focus groups revealed a concern with the concept of 'performance', both in terms of their physical fitness but also, more light-heartedly, in terms of sexual activity.

Campaign design

By taking account of these fragments of knowledge, we were able to construct a campaign which comprehensively engaged its target group and achieved some impressive results. Beginning with the notion of a 'sporting contest' we devised the idea of 'works teams' competing for the championship of a county-wide league over a 6-month 'season'. Points were awarded to individual team members for monthly reductions in percentage body fat (measured by means of a Bodystat device) and aggregated to give a score for the team as a whole.

Prior to the start of the competition (and again at the end of the 6-month period) all team members were given a fitness screening which included a 'Fi-tec' step test, blood pressure test and height/weight recording. As part of their involvement, many participants also completed a Health Education Authority *Look After Yourself* (LAY) course (other workplaces made alternative local arrangements). The LAY course encourages people to build more exercise into their daily lives whilst also providing education about nutrition and stress management. In order to alleviate anxieties about being in the company of more 'sporty types', team membership was limited to those aged between 40 and 55, who had a BMI (body mass index) of more than 27.

Objectives of the campaign

The *Keeping It Up* campaign has three objectives:

1. to influence positively the lifestyles of those in the competing teams
2. to use the participants as 'messengers' who will, in turn, influence friends, relatives and colleagues
3. to generate local publicity about the importance of a healthy lifestyle in the prevention of CHD.

From the beginning of the 1995 campaign, it was also our intention to carry out a comprehensive evaluation of these objectives. The remainder of this chapter presents the most salient findings of the evaluation process.

Introduction to evaluation

We measured both physiological and psychological changes in participants, as well as seeking views about the process and infrastructure of the campaign itself. We did not simply concentrate on those who did well – we also included in the evaluation those who dropped out of the campaign, as well as trying to establish why some employers who were approached decided not to get involved in the first place.

From the outset, there was a strong feeling in the HealthWorks team that we had hit on a model that would work. We wanted to use the process of evaluation as a way of refining and improving the campaign so that it could be repeated in future years.

Involvement of workplaces

Wherever possible, our initial approach to workplaces was made on the basis of existing links with the local (locality-based) Health Promotion Coordinator (HPC). Inevitably, this led to an emphasis on public sector employers in the first running of the campaign. (The second *Keeping It Up* campaign was significantly more successful in engaging private sector employers.) Employers who turned down the opportunity to participate did so, by and large, for administrative reasons, rather than because of any rooted objection to the principle of using the workplace as a base for health promotion. Several employers allowed the *Keeping It Up* exercise and education sessions to be held at least partly in work time – a concession which was warmly welcomed by participants and helped generate a feeling of involvement and support.

Level of participation

Six workplaces fielding a total of nine teams took part in the 1995 campaign. Altogether, 66 men were involved. The only participants to drop out were the small number who had to do so for reasons of injury (not, incidentally, injuries sustained as a result of their participation in the campaign). The reasons most commonly cited for motivation to continue on the programme were:

- the peer support engendered by the competitive nature of the campaign
- a recognition of the health benefits for the individual concerned.

The majority of participants attached great value to the practical instruction in exercise and relaxation techniques. Some teams even made local arrangements to continue to meet as a group after the organised sessions associated with the competition had come to an end.

Many individuals identified changes in the lifestyles of their family as a result of the knowledge they had acquired by participating in the campaign – although there was felt to be rather less impact on nonparticipating work colleagues. Indeed rather regrettably, some participants reported they had become the butt of workplace humour. Of 25 individuals who completed the LAY course and responded to the questionnaire, no fewer than 23 felt unequivocally that their health had benefited from what they had learned.

Administration

Administratively the campaign progressed fairly smoothly, although there were a number of glitches, as might perhaps be expected in a country-wide event such as this, organised for the first time. From the point of view of the HealthWorks team the most difficult part logistically was the coordination of the monthly body fat tests. (It was important for the compilation of the league table that these took place during the same week each month.)

All competitors received a monthly newsletter which aimed to keep them up-to-date with what was happening in the competition – especially with regard to the the current league table. (During the second *Keeping It Up* campaign, the newsletter was more professionally produced and delivered, additionally, a range of other health-related information.) At the end of the competition a ceremony was held at the workplace of the winning team at which the championship trophy was presented. A personal trophy was presented to the individual who had lost the most weight (not, incidentally, a member of the winning team).

Physical outcomes for individual participants

Almost three-quarters of participants showed a reduction in their BMI over the duration of the campaign, and 58% increased their physical fitness as measured by the Fi-tec step test. Almost half showed a reduction in percentage body fat from the beginning to the end of the 6-month period. (However, wide fluctuations in some individual cases during the course of the competition suggest that body fat measurements are not an especially reliable index, except under carefully controlled conditions.) Use of the Bodystat process proved to be a marvellously 'male' way of engaging the interest of participants, combining high-tech gadgetry with immediate statistical evidence of change.

Attitudinal changes in participants

All participants were asked to complete questionnaires at the beginning and end of the competition, to allow us to measure shifts in knowledge, attitude and behaviour. In terms of the links between exercise and health, most participants actually started out with a fairly good knowledge of the facts and knew what they should be concerned about. Few, however, were acting on what they knew, suggesting the presence of that element of denial which many health professionals anecdotally associate with men.

Around half of participants reported that they had increased levels of physical activity in their daily lives as a consequence of their involvement in the campaign. There were some significant increases in knowledge on the subject of nutrition too. Interestingly, almost two-thirds of the men also reported reductions in levels of personal stress.

Longer-term influence of participation

A follow-up questionnaire sent out to all participants 8 months after the end of the competition showed very encouraging results: a majority of respondents had maintained or improved their weight loss. There were similarly positive responses in terms of increased levels of physical activity and greater awareness of the importance of eating healthily. In all, over 80% of respondents agreed with the proposition that they had adopted a healthier lifestyle as a result of their involvement with the *Keeping It Up* campaign.

Conclusions

It is axiomatic in the field of health promotion that establishing the success of an initiative is rarely straightforward. However, there are good grounds for drawing encouraging conclusions from the experience of designing and running the *Keeping It Up* campaign.

In particular, the evaluation of the first programme very strongly confirmed the success of those elements in the campaign which were based on the focus groups we had originally held in the spring of 1995. This is also evidenced more directly by the low dropout rate amongst participants. These elements, of course, were specific to working with men in general and men in this age group in particular. Most notable amongst them were:

- the sporting character of the campaign
- the emphasis on improved performance rather than improved health
- the cameraderie generated by team membership.

There is little doubt in the minds of the HealthWorks team that this model does manage to tap into an essentially male way of looking at the world. In some ways in fact, the development process of this campaign has been more significant than its content and is, in our view, the primary reason for the engagement of a difficult target group.

This is not to say that the outcomes are not important. There is good evidence that many participants not only lost weight and improved their fitness during the course of the programme, but also that a fair proportion of them sustained those gains over subsequent months. It seems too that many participants made attitudinal changes which may form the basis for more positive thinking about their health in the longer term.

These outcomes were achieved by recognising the importance of working in a way which reflects male needs, attitudes and aspirations. We have become accustomed in recent years to the presence of a powerful women's health lobby and the consequent (and rightful) assimilation into the health mainstream of policies which take particular account of women's needs. The absence of a mirror-image men's health lobby may reflect male ambivalence about health (the denial which we have already mentioned). It may also signify a reluctance amongst men to identify 'men's issues' in a more general way. We should not, however, allow the absence of such a lobby and such a tradition to blind us to the need to target health promotion interventions where they are most needed. Men, whether middle-aged, old or young, have specific (and in many cases, very pressing) health needs and we can only work with them successfully by devising strategies which are empathetic.

Key issues for practitioners

- In order to influence men in their 40s and 50s to look after themselves it was vital to find out their opinions. The campaign work undertaken by HealthWorks was based on this research.
- Men rationalise the health risks of an inactive lifestyle, know little about nutrition and diet, and regard exercise as boring. They like competition and team sports.

Practical pointers

- Men were positive about this weight loss programme, because they were part of a workplace team competing against other teams.
- A monthly newsletter helped keep all the men informed of their and others' progress.
- It is vital to design interventions which reflect men's needs, aspirations and attitudes.

13

Alive and Kicking: using sport to improve men's health

Maggie Robinson

Introduction

The Community Education Development Centre (CEDC) is a charitable trust based in Coventry dedicated to widening opportunities for learning. Increasingly, we have been working in the field of health, recognising that working with people in communities is the most effective way of encouraging learning about health.

Up to 1994 CEDC had been working mainly with women and families on projects and consultancies to encourage better access to services and user involvement. The West Midlands

1994 *Report on Public Health*, with its emphasis on the early death and illness of men, dramatically shifted our emphasis. We understood as never before the importance of finding routes into men's lives which would help them improve their own health. We felt particularly strongly that what was needed was development work with young men to raise their awareness of health issues and to assist them to develop healthy lifestyles.

Young men's health in Coventry

At this point we were lucky enough to obtain a small grant from Coventry Health Promotion's community budget to undertake a survey about young men's attitude to health and health services. A group of Coventry workers who had day-to-day contact with individual young men came together for a meeting, at which the concerns about young men's health were outlined. The group decided that a small-scale sample of in-depth interviews would be a cost-effective and practicable way of finding out about young men's attitudes to health in general, to their own health in particular, as well as gauging their knowledge of health and services. The group came up with some ideas about how these interviews should be conducted, and CEDC devised an interviewing schedule.

The interviews were carried out by the workers, either with individuals or with groups. Twenty-seven interviews were carried out in the following group settings:

- in a Moderate Learning Difficulties (MLD) school
- in a Further Education (FE) College
- in a sixth form
- amongst young male volunteers from the Youth Alcohol Project of the Alcohol Advisory Service
- amongst young men using the Coventry Cyrenians
- amongst students at Coventry University.

The ages of the interviewees ranged from 16 to 29.

What is health?

The young men interviewed were given a sheet (see Fig. 13.1) and were asked to put a ring around the six words which had most to do with health, and a cross through the six things which had

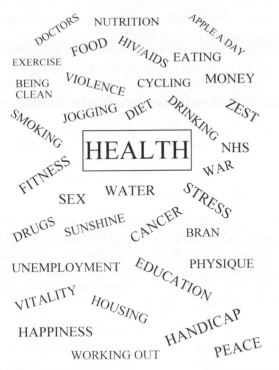

Figure 13.1   Sheet given to young men surveyed to gauge their attitudes to health

least to do with health. What was striking in the results was the emphasis they put on diet and exercise as the basis of health. The ten highest scores were all to do with fitness and diet. This is a constant theme throughout the survey. In most instances, young men equate health with fitness. When asked to comment on what had least to do with health, violence and war scored extremely highly. The impression one is left with is the physicality of men's attitudes to health. This is in marked contrast to the many surveys carried out regarding women's attitudes to health, where relationships and 'happiness' are seen as much more important.

The results of the survey provided some starting points for those working with men in the Coventry project:

■ This emphasis on 'being fit' can be seen as both negative and positive. The following conclusions were drawn:

  − most young men have a different perception of health to that of most young women

- messages about exercise, diet and smoking seem to be having some effect on lifestyle
- more work needs to be done to encourage young men to see health in terms other than the physical
- the young men's preferred contexts of fitness and diet could be used to introduce other facets of health.

■ Young men do think about, and are often concerned about, their health. But asking for advice and help is seen as 'not manly' and embarrassing. Strategies need to be found so that young men can gain support for living a healthy lifestyle, without feeling embarrassment.

■ GPs are recognised by young men as the main source of health advice. This may be based on lack of knowledge about other services, but it would also seem that GPs are seen as an acceptable, factual source of advice and information, whereas 'softer' services such as counsellors and support groups are perceived to be for women.

■ Health advice and information is available through people and services young men feel comfortable with:

- sports teachers
- workers and coaches in leisure centres and sports clubs
- youth club leaders
- managers of training centres
- employers.

The development of *Alive and Kicking*

As a result of our preliminary small-scale research it had become apparent to us, as community educators, that sport was an excellent vehicle by which to reach young men who would otherwise fall through the 'health education' net. We wanted to start with young men where they were (i.e. having an awareness of the 'physicality' of health only), so that we could support them in developing a wider understanding of what health was about.

It is estimated that 35 000 young men play football in the West Midlands. Many of these could be classified as being at risk in the context of their lifestyles. Although it is difficult to describe the average Sunday footballer, research suggests that he:

- is 16–35
- left school at 16
- works in skilled or semi-skilled employment or is unemployed
- may smoke and drink and engage in risk-taking behaviour.

The aims of the project

The main aim of the project was to improve young men's health by working with two Sunday football leagues to raise awareness about healthy lifestyles. We also wanted to:

- enthuse health education and community workers to work with young men to improve their health
- encourage multi-agency approaches
- monitor and evaluate local projects
- disseminate findings nationally.

How the project was implemented

CEDC workers liaised with:

- the secretaries of Coventry and Leicester Sunday football leagues
- Coventry and Leicester health promotion departments
- Coventry City Football Club.

Good relationships were established, and joint working with all three parties was arranged. Coventry Sunday League showed considerable interest, but at the last minute Leicester Football League decided not to take part. The Leamington league was persuaded to take its place. Through League secretaries, CEDC gained information about teams and their organisation. CEDC workers attended preseason meetings of club secretaries to inform them about the project and to get them involved. The League officers were most helpful in supporting our aims and challenging teams to take part.

The project worked in the following way:

- Tasks were sent out to the clubs in one league in each locality. Clubs chosen were in a lowish division in order to target less fit men. The task sheets (see below and Appendix 2) were sent to the club secretaries who were vital to the success of the project.

- In both the Coventry and the Leamington leagues about half the targeted clubs agreed to take part. Each club registered 16 players and 12 clubs took part in the competition, with approximately 200 young men receiving the information and the task sheets in the target age group (18–35-year-olds).

- The tasks were sent out at approximately 2-week intervals and a deadline was given for return, together with a freepost return envelope. Letters and newsletters were sent out together with an updated health league chart.

- A community worker based at CEDC visited clubs, watched games and helped club secretaries to organise the completion of tasks. He reminded secretaries who hadn't returned task sheets and sent out new ones if they had been 'lost'.

- The community worker also obtained and gave out prizes when prize thresholds had been reached.

- Coventry City FC Community Officer visited clubs that took part and offered them free training, which proved popular.

- Although matches were played on a Sunday, most *Alive and Kicking* work was carried out by the teams on their training evening. One of the major tasks was for team members to have a health checkup, and this was carried out by district nurses on training nights at club houses or schools. Nurse facilitators organised the rota of nurses, which worked most successfully in Coventry but not so well in Leamington. This was largely due to the late start in Leamington and illness.

The tasks

The tasks were devised with the help of Coventry Health Promotion Department, which was most supportive, giving us advice and relevant material. Tasks were designed to be of varying difficulty, with differing numbers of points awarded. Some were individual, whilst others encouraged discussion or activity.

Wherever possible they were devised in a football context. Not surprisingly, some were much more successful than others, as the evaluation indicated. There were 10 tasks altogether:

1. Registration and player information
2. Proof of registration with a GP
3. A man's guide to avoiding cancer
4. Alcohol use and abuse
5. Safer sex
6. Healthy eating
7. Send it packing – preparation for No-Smoking Day
8. Spotting the signs – mental health
9. Evaluation of the project
10. Nurse checkups

Two examples of task sheets are shown in Appendix 2.

The competition

As the project was organised in the form of a competition the prizes, league table and prize presentation were important facets. Each team could enter up to 16 players. The completed task sheets were returned to CEDC by the club secretaries in a stamped address envelope provided by us. The sheets were 'marked' and points awarded to the clubs accordingly. The community worker chased up late returns. An updated league chart was sent to the teams with the next set of task sheets.

At agreed points thresholds, clubs were awarded first aid kits and match balls. The club that achieved top marks in each league was awarded a new strip for their team. In liaison with Coventry City FC the top prizes were awarded on the pitch at a premier league game. The presentation was marked by an article in the match programme, which also provided some excellent publicity for Coventry Health Authority's information lines.

Publicity

The project engendered a considerable amount of publicity locally, with several articles in local newspapers, coverage through Coventry City FC, interviews on local radio and a film for Central TV News.

Articles for health professionals have appeared in *The Guardian*, *Healthlines* and *The Young People's Health Network Newsletter*. There have also been articles in CEDC's own magazine *Network*, *Working with Men* and *The Times Educational Supplement*.

The evaluation

The evaluation was carried out internally by means of discussions with workers on the project and with football league personnel. Task 9 gave the men taking part an opportunity to comment on the project. In all, 80 completed the evaluation, though some did not answer all the questions. The results were as follows:

■ Do you think that the *Alive and Kicking* project is:

  – a good idea 63%
  – interesting 54%
  – every club should do it 45%
  – quite a good idea 26%
  – useful 28%
  – enjoyable 21%
  – totally pointless 0%
  – irritating 5%.

(Any number of boxes could be completed, but many respondents only ticked one).

■ The tasks we were given were, on the whole:

  – much too hard 1%
  – much too easy 10%
  – about right 86%.

■ Which tasks did you find most useful?

  – Healthy eating for performance
  – A man's guide to avoiding cancer
  – The health checkup.

■ Which tasks did you find the least useful?

  – Registering with a GP
  – Signing the pledge about drinking over Christmas.

- Has the project changed your lifestyle in any way?
  - not at all 30%
  - slightly 45%
  - definitely 6%.

- What are the areas in which you have made changes?
  - improved diet
  - better protection against skin cancer
  - giving up smoking.

- Do you feel better informed about healthy lifestyles?
  - no 4%
  - slightly 46%
  - definitely 30%.

- Would you recommend the scheme to a friend in another league?
  - Yes 76%
  - No 4%.

- Do you think the prizes were good?
  - Yes 75%.

- Did you find the free training sessions useful?
  - Yes 65%.

Keith Harrison, Manager of the Warwick Sporting Colts team, is certainly positive about the project, as well as being honest about the reasons for his team's participation:

> When we first got involved, our main motivation was to win the equipment. But the lads got into it – nobody refused to take part – and I think the project may have made them more aware of their health and how changing their behaviour could make them fitter for football. We'd definitely do it again, even if there were no prizes!

Key factors to success

The underlying factors to our success include:

- the community education approach
- reaching out to young men where they are most comfortable
- using the strong unit of the football team to motivate young men to participate in the project.

Other vital factors were:

- establishing positive contact with local Football Associations
- meeting and selling the project to league secretaries
- meeting club secretaries at league-organised meetings
- allowing the league to identify the appropriate division
- building relationships with club secretaries
- developing health activities in liaison with local health promotion departments
- active, hands-on project management
- prizes being awarded regularly
- The involvement of the local professional club was useful, but not seen as essential.

Difficulties and limitations

One of the major problems encountered during this project was the difference in style between health services and sports clubs. We carried out most of the work at the weekday evening practice sessions, not on Sunday mornings. Nevertheless, it was difficult for us (and even more so for 'official' health services) to cope with abandoned matches because of weather conditions, and locating changing rooms in unknown schools and playing fields. However, as essentially community educators we are more used to this kind of work than health workers. Having a hands-on community educator was vital to the success of the project.

We were working with men who were already involved in sport, so they were not the least fit group. However, we did choose to work with lower leagues where the men were not so committed to fitness. This meant, though, that some team members were uncommitted and did not always turn up to practice.

There are considerable limitations to working through a sports context, but for men in Britain sport is a very important cultural context. There are few men who are not involved in any kind of sport, be it only as a supporter. Since our project started, we have seen an increasing number of projects based around sport – for example *Kick Out Racism in Sport*. We must be wary of overkill. Working through Sunday morning leagues rather than through league clubs is another approach.

Conclusion

The differing attitudes of health promotion workers towards the project was interesting. Most believed, as we did, that we should start where the young men were, in a situation where they felt relaxed and at home. Others thought, with some justification, that the *Alive and Kicking* approach would only reinforce men's competitive approach to life.

However, despite these concerns, the project does appear to have been successful in reaching young men and, at the very least, raising awareness about healthy lifestyles. The approach is flexible and could be adapted to a number of sports – basketball and pub cricket are two contexts we are interested in exploring. Reaching boys between 8 and 14, when they are developing notions of lifestyles, and when sport is of great interest to many, is our next goal. We are currently setting up health competitions across under-12 football teams in Nuneaton, and in after-school clubs in Carlisle.

From our work with young men in Coventry, and from *Alive and Kicking*, we conclude with the following recommendations:

- Health education delivered by schools and other agencies needs to take young men's perceptions of health into account.

- Young men require advice, information and support delivered in a variety of ways and locations that are relevant to their lives.

- Well-targeted and appropriate marketing and publicity are very important in ensuring that young men have information and support.

- GPs are young men's first choice when they need to seek advice. GP services need to be appropriate for young men.

- From an early age boys should be encouraged to express their feelings and gain experience in communicating their needs in a variety of contexts, such as at the doctor's.

- Health advice is available to young men as part of other services not labelled health.

- Health 'checkups' should be regarded as a national prerequisite to taking part in a variety of activities for young men, for example, joining a sports club.

Key issues for practitioners

- Preliminary research, even on a small scale, is useful in determining appropriate types of intervention.
- Health education needs to take into account young men's perceptions of health – in this case the findings that young men equate health with fitness and that asking for help is seen as embarrassing.
- There is a danger that working through fitness and sport may reinforce men's competitive approach to life.
- Young men require information and advice delivered in a variety of ways and locations.

Practical pointers

- Multiagency working is very important in accessing and sustaining contact with men.
- Competitions and prizes can help sustain men's involvement.
- Using sport and fitness does not reach the most unfit men.
- Well-targeted marketing and publicity is vital to get information to young men.

14

Primary care

David Jewell

This chapter covers:

- causes of male morbidity and mortality
  - cardiovascular disease
  - cancer
  - accidents
  - suicide
- possible explanations
  - biological risks
  - acquired risks
  - pyschosocial aspects
  - health reporting behaviour
  - prior health behaviour
- what can be done in primary care?
  - cardiovascular disease prevention
  - family interventions
  - identifying men with particular needs
  - depression
  - health education
  - organisation of primary care
- key issues for practitioners
- practical pointers.

Introduction

A boy born in England in 1996 can expect to live to the age of 75, 5 years less than a girl. The higher mortality rate for men persists at all ages, but is at a peak in adolescence and early adult life. Yet men are much less visible than women in general practice. The 1991–92 National Morbidity Survey reported consultation rates of 4.2 per year for women, compared with 2.7 for men. The difference is most marked among those aged 25–44, when the rates are 4.3 for women and 1.9 for men (Royal College of General Practitioners, Office of Population Censuses and Surveys, Department of Health, 1995).

The invisibility of men's health is reflected in other ways. It has only recently surfaced as a matter worthy of study, compared with the long (and honourable) history of interest in women's health. So while women's health clinics are commonplace in general practice, services specifically designed to cater for men are the exception rather than the rule. One reason proposed for this is the sociological invisibility of men. Men are seen as being the dominant culture, while women, paradoxically, see themselves as being a minority, or at least a special interest, group. It has, by the same argument, taken a long time for men to see that there is a health agenda that applies to them as men.

This invisibility is matched by ignorance on the part of most doctors, and covers many aspects of illnesses that affect men. To take the most obvious example, there is a striking lack of information on the results of prostate operations on patients' feelings about themselves as men. There do not appear to be any simple solutions to the 'problem' of men's health. What emerges is a complex situation. We need to know much more about the various influences and their interaction before we can be confident about effective interventions.

Causes of male morbidity and mortality

The causes of excess male morbidity and mortality are well known. They include cardiovascular disease, cancer, accidents and suicide. In addition, and apart from conditions such as prostate cancer which are exclusively the province of men, there is a male excess in nonfatal disease in gout, chronic obstructive airways disease, AIDS, duodenal ulcer and inguinal hernia.

Cardiovascular disease

Coronary disease kills about 180 000 people annually in the UK, three-quarters of them men. In the under 50 age group the rate for death of men is six times that of women. Some of this excess is the result of women being protected by female sex hormones. It is now widely recognised that giving hormone replacement therapy to women prolongs their much lower heart disease rate, as long as the hormones are taken.

Modern preoccupation has concentrated on 'lifestyle' risk factors in the origins of cardiovascular disease:

- smoking
- diet
- high blood pressure
- obesity
- lack of exercise.

Certainly smoking is more common in men (although the figures suggesting this excess is much less than it used to be and may at some time in the future disappear). Debate on diet has in the past focused on saturated fat intake, but it is now shifting to intake of particular foods such as fish oils and antioxidants in fruit and vegetables. It is possible that the stereotypical 'male' diet may be lower in such items than the stereotypical 'female' diet. There is no difference between the blood pressures of men and women. In contrast, men tend to take more exercise than women and this should have a protective effect. Obesity is more common in men than in women, but it has been suggested that it is the pattern of obesity that is most important. The central obesity more commonly seen in men is thought to be particularly risky for heart disease compared with peripheral obesity more commonly seen in women (Waldron 1995).

Such risk factors do not explain all the difference between incidence in men and women. In one study in Scotland, after correction for cholesterol levels, smoking, blood pressure, obesity and social class, men aged 60–64 still had twice the mortality rate from ischaemic heart disease as women of the same age (Isles et al 1992). A study in the *British Medical Journal* (Ruston, Clayton & Calnan 1998) has confirmed previous evidence that patients often delay calling the doctor because they fail to recognise chest pain as being the result of myocardial infarction. Men may be particularly at fault here.

Cancer

Mortality rates from both bladder and lung cancer are higher in men than in women. The higher rate in lung cancer is directly attributable to smoking; the only known risk factors for bladder cancer are smoking and certain industrial hazards.

Accidents

Road traffic accidents account for half of all accidental deaths. The remainder are predominantly due to falls, followed by causes such as drowning. All are more common in men, especially in young men under the age of 25, and this is thought to be the result of men's increased willingness to take risks.

Suicide

One particularly puzzling piece of data is the considerably larger number of deaths from suicide among men. Since 1911 there has been an excess among men, and the rates in men and women ran parallel until 1975. From then until 1990 the rates diverged: rates among men rose, while among women they fell (Charlton et al 1992). The mortality data for 1998 record four times as many suicides among men as among women (2826 and 788 respectively). These rates (109 per million for men; 30 per million for women) were very similar to those in Europe as a whole (Office for National Statistics 1999).

The puzzle is that rates of depression among men have been shown in both community surveys and clinical data to be lower among men that among women. Again the suggestion is that men react differently to life's stresses: women express their distress more openly and present more commonly to doctors; men externalise theirs as aggression and antisocial activity (Paykel 1991).

Possible explanations

In a major review of the influences of gender on health, Verbrugge (1985) explored five different explanations for the imbalance in health:

1. biological risks
2. acquired risks
3. psychological aspects

4. health reporting behaviour
5. prior health behaviour.

These are examined below.

Biological risks

It is clear that at least some of the protection that women have from heart disease is biological, mediated by circulating oestrogen. Apart from this, and the diseases experienced exclusively by men, it is difficult to ascribe much of the difference to simple biological differences.

Acquired risks

Men's higher rates of smoking and alcohol intake increase their risk of lung cancer and chronic obstructive airways disease, and may also be responsible for higher rates of duodenal ulcer, and for some of the higher rates of cardiovascular disease. Men are exposed to greater risks from work and sport. Women are believed to use more behaviours to protect themselves against hazards in everyday life. These include varying their daily activities and turning to others for support. In this they are using stronger emotional ties to others as a buffer against disease. Research has suggested that friendship between women is more emotionally supportive than that between men, where there is more likely to be shared activity than emotional intimacy.

Psychosocial aspects

In all aspects of illness behaviour women are seen to be 'better' patients than men. They are more sensitive to bodily discomfort; more likely to evaluate their symptoms as related to physical illness; more willing to take action, both using lay networks and consulting professionals. Women are better at complying with agreed regimes of medicine taking, using sickness absence and follow-up visits to doctors. It is likely that the different ways in which they have been socialised as children, and the different roles that they adopt as adults, particularly in relation to children, influence men and women in this area.

Health reporting behaviour

Women are better at remembering and disclosing information about their health. There is the intriguing suggestion that some of this behaviour may be related to the different ways in which men and women use language, a subject that has been extensively researched in other fields.

Prior health behaviour

Experience of the sick role can change perceptions. Good experiences of illness and medical care are likely to improve trust in services and encourage future disclosure of health problems.

What can be done in primary care?

Given this very brief summary of the state of men's health, what can general practice set out to do to address the problems? At risk of being too nihilistic, it is important to acknowledge two limiting factors at the outset:

1. Clearly some of the differences (those attributable to biological influences) can never be changed. Many of the others are attributable to the ways in which men are socialised, and it is important to be realistic about how quickly this is likely to be amenable to any change.
2. There is a suspicion that the way that general practice is organised makes it more difficult for men to deal with health problems. Both the siting and the timing of general practice availability make it more difficult for those working to consult their doctors.

To any casual observer, primary care staff are now overwhelmingly female, with male general practitioners being the exception among the large numbers of nurses, health visitors, and receptionists. Large numbers of contacts focus around women's health agenda, and the needs of children are, even now, much more frequently handled by mothers than by fathers. This may mean that general practice is seen as a female domain. There is intuitive sense in the idea of providing healthcare in settings where people spend their time. For men this could include youth clubs for adolescents, or workplace settings for adult men.

Comparison with other programmes and services provided for women is instructive in demonstrating, as much as anything else, the influence of time. For instance, the cervical cancer screening programme started being set up many years ago and the breast cancer screening programme more recently (1991).

In both cases considerable doubt has been expressed about whether the programmes can deliver the health gains that were originally intended (Gøtzsche & Olsen 2000). In contrast, the question of using Prostate Specific Antigen in a screening programme for early diagnosis and treatment of prostate cancer has arisen only recently. With the experience of previous screening programmes, the Department of Health has made it clear that it has no intention of introducing such a programme without sound evidence of benefit. Proposals for studies are currently being planned to provide such evidence.

For testicular cancer the idea of testicular self-examination has been proposed. Again there is doubt that promoting regular self-examination (as opposed to leaving it up to the men to detect swellings by chance, as they have done up till now) will have any benefit. However many observers treat the idea with some amusement, doubting that men would even take this seriously. The contrast with the way that breast awareness is promoted demonstrates the difference in the way men and women are seen to approach health matters.

Given these limitations, it is nevertheless possible to identify a range of initiatives that general practice could undertake to address a specific agenda for men's health.

Cardiovascular disease prevention

Following the success of 'well woman' clinics, some practices have set up 'well man' clinics, primarily in order to offer screening for cardiovascular risk factors. Such initiatives have not been widely copied, partly at least as a result of the publication of two large studies in the UK which have questioned the value of multiphasic primary prevention of cardiovascular disease for both men and women (Family Heart Study Group 1994, Imperial Cancer Research Fund OXCHECK Study Group 1994).

As hopes for primary prevention of cardiovascular disease have faltered, attention has turned towards secondary prevention, where the purpose is to prevent further disease in those who are already affected by disease. One study from Northern Ireland reported success in this area using intermediate outcomes (Cupples & McKnight 1994). However, this has not been confirmed by a larger study in southern England (Jolly et al 1999). The conventional explanation is that in people who are at highest risk of further disease there is the potential for the greatest benefit. However, they may also be the most highly motivated to undertake the lifestyle changes required. This is one hint of what may make a programme effective.

Cardiac rehabilitation among those recovering from myocardial infarctions is one intervention that has been well researched. This includes programmes of graded exercise intended to improve the cardiac fitness of participants. The benefits include:

- increased physical fitness
- reduced blood pressure
- weight loss
- psychological benefit
- improved chance of return to work
- improved survival (Bethell 1998).

Exercise programmes are unusual among health programmes in that men are more likely than women to enrol, and less likely to withdraw (McGee and Horgan 1992). Their success provides further clues about what may or may not work in the future: they are likely to take place in centres associated with sport rather than health and disease and may be overseen by sportsmen rather than doctors and nurses. A recent survey found less than half of existing programmes included a physician on the rehabilitation team (Lewin et al 1998). Finally, of course, exercise is consistent with conventional notions of masculinity.

Family interventions

It is ironic that those professing to call themselves family doctors so rarely see whole families. It is commonplace to see children with one parent, and older patients with a younger carer. However, seeing couples together is unusual, even when there is an explicit relationship problem being presented.

However, the role of families in determining lifestyles, establishing patterns of illness behaviour, and supporting or undermining attempts to change lifestyle, is well known (Wilson 1998). Handling family problems is not a standard part of most general practitioners' training. Willingness, or insistence on seeing partners as a couple may be a more effective way of helping, but it may also convey a powerful educational message that the emotional agenda is the responsibility of both men and women. In particular, general practitioners can encourage men to take responsibility for their own health, rather than, as so many still do, leaving their partners to do the worrying for them.

Identifying men with particular needs

Research evidence shows that the most vulnerable groups of men are those recently widowed, separated or divorced (Jewell 1998). Those who have never married are also at increased risk of cardiovascular disease. It is not clear what action will be effective in preventing death or serious disease in these groups, but a small amount of additional attention is unlikely to do any harm and may provide support and the opportunity to discuss their feelings.

Other groups of men have particular needs, but may be difficult to reach. They include adolescent boys, men under threat of or undergoing redundancy, and the recently retired. Such groups may indicate a need for a more proactive approach, such as offering help by running group sessions that don't have illness as a prerequisite.

Depression

In recent years numerous studies have shown that depression is often not identified by general practitioners, and a lot of effort has been devoted to improving this aspect of primary care. The reasons that have been suggested include:

- poor training of general practitioners
- lack of time to explore difficult areas
- patients' tendency to somatise their symptoms and their unwillingness to recognise the symptoms as having psychological origin.

Men are widely believed to have particular difficulty acknowledging mental distress and may be especially prone to somatise. It is possible that this explains some, but probably not all, of the lower rates of depression recorded among men. It seems sensible for general practitioners to remember this when all men consult, and to develop sensitive skills of exploring mental distress in men unwilling to acknowledge it.

Health education

Accepting the arguments about men's greater reluctance to consult and then follow the advice of doctors, and the consequences of this for their health, then it is clear that general practitioners have a duty to influence men's illness behaviour. In their seminal paper, Stott & Davis (1979) pointed out that every consultation offers opportunities other than dealing with the presenting complaint. This doesn't mean long educational sessions, but limited exchange of views and information intended to bring about small incremental changes in men's illness behaviour. Such activity can be supplemented with printed information.

This is, of course, unlikely to bring about sudden and major change in men's patterns of behaviour. However, as with the issue of smoking, doctors are working within a context and can make a small contribution to a wider social change. Bozett and Forester (1989) have suggested the need for a 'men's health nurse practitioner' to answer some of the longer term needs of men.

Organisation of primary care

In England, all practices became members of Primary Care Groups on 1 April 1999, as set out in the White Paper published in December 1997 (Secretary of State for Health 1997). Primary Care Groups are currently deciding whether to take on the independent status and more onerous duties of becoming Primary Care Trusts (PCTs). At this early stage it is impossible to predict how they will develop or how they will influence the development of primary care in the future. At one extreme is the pessimistic view, that PCTs will become the bodies responsible for making difficult rationing decisions made more difficult by trying to hold the ring between practices at odds with each other. At the other is the optimistic one, which envisages PCTs having the resources and expertise to assess local needs and set up innovative models of collaborative healthcare for vulnerable groups. After the contract written for Primary Care in 1966, it took many years for general practitioners to make full use of the opportunities offered. It seems almost certain that it will take as long for practices to learn to work together and make the best use of the new opportunities offered by this, probably much more radical, change.

Conclusion

If the above constitutes the sum total of what primary care might be offering in the future, then it does not amount to much. If all this activity were happening it might not be visible as 'Men's Health Services'. The gloomy conclusion might be that conventional primary care has little to offer men, and that effective advances will have to take place elsewhere.

Primary care, both in the UK and elsewhere, is a conservative discipline reflecting the culture in which it operates. The widespread setting-up of well woman clinics in Britain was not only a convenient way of dealing with an obvious set of physical problems by what was at the time a largely male-staffed profession. It was also an expression of a sociopolitical movement drawing attention to the particular needs of women. Likewise, in its provision of services for men, primary care will not lead but will follow. The major advance will be in helping men to be more sensitive to their own health needs. This debate will take time, and general practitioners will have their own contribution to make. Only then will they begin to understand how to answer men's health needs.

Key issues for practitioners

- A review of men's health issues suggests that we need to know more about the various influences and their interactions before we can be sure of what constitute effective interventions.

- The opportunities for interventions in primary care are limited: the organisation of general practice makes it more difficult for men to deal with health problems. It may be that effective advances will have to take place elsewhere.

Practical pointers

- Men are more likely to take notice of health information away from the primary care setting e.g. in sport and fitness venues.
- It may be effective for GPs to see men with their partners, as a couple.

References

Bethell H J N 1998 Cardiovascular disease. In: O'Dowd T, Jewell D (eds) Men's health. Oxford University Press, Oxford, pp 221–238

Bozett F W, Forester D A 1989 A proposal for a men's health nurse practitioner. IMAGE: Journal of Nursing Scholarship, 21:158–161

Charlton J, Kelly S, Dunnell K, Evans B, Jenkins R, Wallis R 1992 Trends in suicide deaths in England and Wales. Population Trends 69:10–16

Cupples M E, McKnight A 1994 Randomised controlled trial of health promotion in general practice for patients at high cardiovascular risk. British Medical Journal 309:993–996

Family Heart Study Group 1994 Randomised controlled trial evaluating cardiovascular screening and intervention in general practice: principal results of the British Family Heart Study. British Medical Journal 308:313–320

Gøtzsche P C, Olsen O 2000 Is screening for breast cancer with mammography justifiable? Lancet 355:129–134

Imperial Cancer Research Fund OXCHECK Study Group 1994 Effectiveness of health checks conducted by nurses in primary care: results of the OXCHECK study after one year. British Medical Journal 308:308–312

Isles C G, Hole D J, Hawthorne V M, Lever A F 1992 Relation between coronary risk and coronary mortality in women of the Renfrew and Paisley survey: comparison with men. Lancet 339:702–706

Jewell D 1998 Adult life. In: O'Dowd T, Jewell D (eds) Men's health. Oxford University Press, Oxford, pp 45–60

Jolly K, Bradley F, Sharp S, Smith H, Thompson S, Kinmonth A-L, Mant D for the SHIP collaborative group 1999 Randomised controlled trial of follow up care in general practice of patients with myocardial infarction and angina: final results of the Southampton Heart Integrated Care Project (SHIP). British Medical Journal 318:706–711

Lewin R J P, Ingleton R, Newens A J, Thompson D R 1998 Adherence to cardiac rehabilitation guidelines: a survey of rehabilitation programmes in the United Kingdom. British Medical Journal 316:1354–1355

McGee H M, Horgan J H 1992 Cardiac rehabilitation programmes: are women less likely to attend? British Medical Journal 305:283–284

Office for National Statistics 1999 Mortality statistics. Review of the Registrar General on deaths by cause, sex and age in England and Wales 1998. HMSO, London

Paykel E S 1991 Depression in women. British Journal of Psychiatry 158(suppl 10):22–29

Royal College of General Practitioners, Office of Population Censuses and Surveys, Department of Health 1995 Morbidity statistics from general practice. Fourth national study 1991–1992. HMSO, London

Ruston A, Clayton J, Calnan M 1998 Patients' action during their cardiac event: qualitative study exploring differences and modifiable factors. British Medical Journal 316:1060–1065

Secretary of State for Health 1997 The new NHS. Modern. Dependable. The Stationery Office, London

Stott N C H and Davis R H 1979 The exceptional potential of every primary care consultation. Journal of the Royal College of General Practitioners 29:201–205

Verbrugge L 1985 Gender and health: an update on hypothesis and evidence. Journal of Health and Social Behaviour 26:156–182

Waldron I 1995 Contributions of biological and behavioural factors to changing sex differences in ischaemic heart disease mortality. In: Lopez A D, Caselli G, Valkonen T (eds) Adult mortality in developed countries: from description to explanation. Clarendon Press, Oxford

Wilson A 1998 Getting help. In: O'Dowd T, Jewell D (eds) Men's health. Oxford University Press, Oxford, pp 259–271

15

Well Man Clinics

Christine Watson

Introduction

This chapter describes the experience of the Department of Family Planning and Reproductive Health Care of Optimum Health Services NHS Trust (since incorporated into Community Health South London NHS Trust) in setting up a Well Man Clinic to serve the inner London boroughs of Lewisham and North Southwark.

Background

Our motivation to open a Well Man Clinic was originally triggered in the early 1980s by some of our female clients in family planning and Well Woman Clinics, who asked us why we did not provide a parallel service for their partners. Although in theory our family planning services were targeted at both sexes, very few men registered as clients and our Well Woman Clinics had been developed to provide a holistic service targeted exclusively at women, generally those who were not currently needing family planning advice (Watson 1989).

We were already well aware of the differential mortality of men and women in our district (Stevens 1987) and our plans to develop a service for men were given further impetus in the report of the Chief Medical Officer for 1992, which highlighted the disproportionate mortality and morbidity experienced by British men over a wide range of diseases (Calman 1993).

Similar initiatives

Around 1984 we had become aware of a number of initiatives in men's health. A Well Man Clinic had been opened in Castlemilk, Glasgow by two male health visitors. Also in 1984 the Family Planning Association (FPA) launched its *Men Too* campaign, which had been accompanied by the publication of *Men, Sex and Contraception* (Birth Control Trust & Family Planning Association 1984). In 1985 two male district nurses opened the first male family planning clinic in North Manchester and a Well Man Clinic was opened in Brent (Pownall 1985). Our ambition to open our own clinic was frustrated at that time by a lack of resources, but by 1994 we had identified sufficient savings from our family planning budget to set up a pilot service.

Planning and implementation

We convened a small planning group of eight people (male and female) which included the following:

- a senior health promotion adviser
- a general practitioner
- a development coordinator for Brook (Youth) Advisory Centres
- a nurse training coordinator
- administrative, nursing and medical staff from the department of Family Planning and Reproductive Health Care.

The group met on three occasions between January and March 1994. Our aims were:

- to review previous initiatives in providing Well Men services
- to identify health resources already on offer to men locally
- to identify what health services for men could complement existing local provision
- to determine when, where and how such services might be provided.

We concluded that it would be difficult to attract men to any health promotion service, but that we should make an attempt. There was little in the way of targeted services for men in the Lewisham area and while there were a number of ongoing youth projects in south-east London, there was little provision for men in older age groups. We therefore decided to target the age group 20–65, and to open a facility in Lewisham.

We felt that we would need to recruit and train motivated staff who would be able to offer counselling, assessment, management and/or referral for a wide range of needs including:

- contraception
- reproductive and sexual health
- maturational and relationship problems
- substance misuse
- mental health problems
- medical problems
- lifestyle issues.

We decided to call the clinic *Open for Men* hoping that this would indicate a welcoming and open-ended approach. Although the service was to be targeted at men, it was felt that female partners should not be excluded if couples wished to attend together. After considering Saturday morning as a possible time for our single weekly session, we finally decided that Friday evening from 6.30 to 9 pm was a more promising time. We were able to secure premises in a central Lewisham community clinic, well served by public transport.

Following the family planning and Well Woman Clinic model we originally planned a multidisciplinary staff team including a receptionist, a nurse and a doctor who would all have received family planning training. We suspected that a nonmedical counsellor would be a welcome addition to the team and were fortunate to obtain the services of a voluntary counsellor, 3 months after the clinic opened. It was felt that the staff did not need to be exclusively men, but that male staff should always be available. When recruitment was complete the staff team comprised the following members:

- receptionist (female)
- nurse (two males job-sharing)
- doctor (female)
- counsellor (male).

In advance of the clinic opening, the following items of stationery were designed and printed, in order to record activity and assist in evaluating the clinic:

- a semistructured male casenote system
- a patient checklist (see Table 15.1, p. 170)
- a statistical record sheet ('the clinic session sheet').

A wide range of health promotion leaflets relevant to men's health was identified and ordered and a staff dossier was compiled containing information on evidence-based approaches to men's health issues such as testicular or prostatic cancer, and helping clients with tobacco or alcohol addiction.

Publicity for the new service was carefully planned and considerable efforts were made to distribute posters, flyers and other publicity material via the following:

- women partners attending our existing family planning and Well Woman Clinics
- general practitioners
- genitourinary medicine clinics
- local employers and job centres
- libraries
- health service premises
- pubs and clubs
- local radio and newspapers.

Publicity emphasised the following aspects of the clinic:

- free, personal and confidential
- timed appointments available via a central booking service
- clients could also 'walk in' without appointments
- the wide range of services on offer
- male staff always available.

The clinic eventually opened in September 1994. There was the possibility that no-one would attend – or that we would be overwhelmed as a result of our extensive publicity. In fact, a reasonable number of men came right from the start, and although numbers have gradually increased they remain manageable.

Staff management

Line management and professional supervision have been provided by managers in the Department of Family Planning and Reproductive Health Care and, for the counsellor, by an experienced freelance supervisor. The staff attended a formal meeting with management on a 6-monthly basis during the first 3 years, after which it was felt that once a year was sufficient. At this meeting, working practices and statistics are reviewed and training needs agreed. Initial orientation training for the staff has been followed by relevant inservice training and updating. All the clinical staff have received additional training and have ongoing supervision in the management of sexual problems, as this was identified as one of the main client needs. Liaison with the local mental health services, including those for substance misuse, has been fostered and self-help materials are provided in the clinic for clients suffering from depression, anxiety or phobic disorders.

Clinic activity

Figures from the time the clinic opened on 2 September 1994 to 31 March 1999 show that during that period, 751 men had registered with *Open for Men*. Approximately 150 new clients present in each financial year and annual attendances have varied between 400 and 500. On average three new clients attend each session with an additional six making return visits.

Clients have proved to be keen to make and keep appointments. During the first financial year of operation 323 (84%) of the 385 appointments were kept, while a further 83 clients 'walked in' opportunistically.

The majority of clients were local residents and about a third identified themselves as members of minority ethnic groups. There has been an observable shift in the age distribution. In

1995–96 the largest 10-year cohort was aged 25–34, but in 1996–97 it was 35–44. The clinic has therefore achieved its aim of attracting men past their teenage years.

When clients first arrive, they are registered by the clinic receptionist. They are asked to give their name, date of birth, address and the name of their general practitioner, although the latter would not be informed of the client's attendance without prior consent.

Clients are then invited to complete a questionnaire. The aim of this is to demonstrate that the staff are open to discuss a very wide range of issues and to allow clients one or more starting points for an interview. The reasons for attending given by new clients over four consecutive quarters from 1 October 1994 to 30 September 1995 are shown in Table 15.1. The most popular

Table 15.1   Replies to questionnaires completed by 164 of 168 consecutive new clients (1 October 1994–30 September 1995)

Reason for attending	No. of clients	% of clients
Free condoms	42	25.6
Information on safer sex or HIV/AIDS	20	12.2
Information on sexually transmitted infections	16	9.8
General contraceptive advice	13	7.9
Information on vasectomy	12	7.3
Sexual or relationship problems	46	28.0
My physical development	25	15.2
Getting or keeping fit	43	26.2
Being fertile	9	5.5
Planning to be a parent	12	7.3
Health problems	51	31.1
Stress, depression or anxiety	48	29.3
Bereavement	6	3.7
Violence	6	3.7
Alcohol	10	6.1
Drugs	3	1.8
Giving up smoking	18	11.0
A health check – a personal MOT	99	60.4
How to look after my health	39	23.8
Anything else? If so, please describe.	11	6.7
TOTAL	529*	

*Total exceeds 164 as more than one reason was usually listed

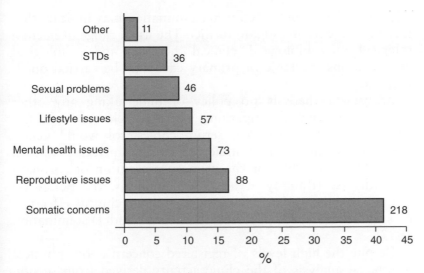

Figure 15.1 **Summary and classification of 529 requests for help (1 October 1994–30 September 1995)**

was 'a health check'. Figure 15.1 represents an attempt to classify and rank these reasons. It should be noted that clients frequently indicated more than one reason for attending. Somatic concerns can be seen to predominate, accounting for 218 (41%) of the 529 responses. These are followed in rank order by reproductive issues, mental health issues, lifestyle issues, sexual problems, sexually transmitted infections and other concerns.

Clients can choose whether they see the counsellor, the nurse, the doctor or more than one member of these. At some point, most clients will undergo a routine medical history which includes enquiries about general health, family history, social history and a sexual, reproductive and contraceptive history. An initial examination is also offered which includes recording of:

- weight
- height
- blood pressure
- urine analysis for glucose, albumen and nitrites
- clinical examination of the chest, abdomen and genitalia, taking the opportunity to teach testicular self-examination.

Factors in the history or clinical examination may indicate that it is advisable to investigate further. The usual range of haematological, microbiological, clinical chemistry and radiological investigations available in primary care may be carried out if required.

At present there is no policy of undertaking any other routine screening investigations where no clear benefit has been shown. For example, serum cholesterol would generally only be measured if indicated by the corrected version of the Sheffield table for the primary prevention of coronary heart disease (Ramsay et al 1996). Similarly, the policy on testing for prostate specific antigen follows clinical effectiveness guidelines (NHS Centre for Reviews and Dissemination 1997).

Despite the high levels of registered concern about physical health, an analysis of the clinic activity derived from session sheets completed by the staff reveals that most clients are offered help within the clinic. The services provided include:

- counselling on a wide range of issues
- provision of condoms and teaching their correct use
- counselling about other contraceptive methods (e.g. vasectomy) or safe sex
- subfertility investigation
- advice on anxiety management or other mental health problems
- lifestyle advice on stress, exercise, diet, alcohol, drugs or smoking
- specific psychological or physical treatments for sexual dysfunction.

The nonmedical counsellor is able to take on some clients for longer term counselling and this has been found to be helpful for clients with relationship difficulties, bereavement problems and maturational anxieties.

The staff have found that although physical symptoms are often presented initially, once clients are assured of time and confidentiality, more profound concerns may be disclosed. There is a clinical impression (which needs to be tested objectively) that men need longer consultation times than women in order to get to the 'heart of the matter'. This may be an underlying reason for the high rate of return visits.

Table 15.2   **External referrals (1 April 1995–31 March 1996)**

Identified problem	Clients (n=161)	%
Genitourinary medicine	13	8.1
Urology	3	1.9
Hypertension	7	4.3
Sexual/relationship problem	5	3.1
Alcohol misuse	1	0.6
Mental health	2	1.2
Other medical problems	20	12.4
TOTAL	51	

Although clients have been helped with most of their problems within the clinic, some assessments have resulted in referral to other services for further treatment. During the first full financial year of operation (1995–96), when 161 registered clients made 406 visits, onward referrals were made 51 times, with some men being referred to more than one agency. Conditions such as previously undiagnosed hypertension, diabetes mellitus, clinical depression and sexually transmitted diseases were detected, presenting the opportunity for therapeutic intervention (see Table 15.2).

Difficulties

Initial difficulties setting up this clinic revolved around finding the necessary funding and a suitable venue. We were able to free up the necessary financial resources by closing a weekly family planning session which was underused and where it was judged that existing clients could transfer to alternative provision without undue hardship – although this inevitably attracted some criticism. In order to secure the use of one of our existing clinics during unsocial hours (Friday evenings) we had to make a strong case to our management colleagues and agree that our clinical staff would be responsible for the security of the building, to avoid the additional expense of caretaking. This falls short of the ideal.

Since the clinic has been operational, we have encountered few difficulties. The potential security problem has not manifested itself to any great extent. Our female receptionist has been provided with a personal alarm with which she can quickly summon the assistance of her colleagues, but she has never used it. There have been a few inappropriate referrals to the clinic; most men are self-referred and the staff have felt confident in offering them help.

The clinic premises are not entirely satisfactory, particularly because the soundproofing between consulting rooms and the waiting room is poor. While we wait for this to be remedied, staff have to speak quietly and encourage clients to do likewise, in order to fulfil our commitment to confidentiality. We have tried playing music in the waiting room but this has proved distracting and it is difficult to please all tastes!

Fulfilling the commitment to giving each client sufficient time when they need it is probably the greatest challenge. Appointments are set at 15-minute intervals to cope with client demand but consultations can last for 20–30 minutes and sometimes waiting times build up. Teamwork and effective consultation skills are seen as the key to overcoming this difficulty.

Successful features

We feel that we were fortunate in being able to recruit an excellent and dedicated staff team who have worked extremely well together. We were also gratified that we seemed to have predicted the range of needs with a fair degree of accuracy. Practitioners wishing to set up their own services would be well advised to conduct a needs assessment exercise and plan staff recruitment and training around this before launching. Careful monitoring by the staff can help to ensure that basic activity data are recorded to support the case for continued funding.

The future

This innovative service remains viable and may prove to be a useful model for similar services in inner city locations. Before this happens, further research should be conducted to examine the cost-effectiveness, qualitative aspects, health outcomes and consumer views of the clinic.

Key issues for practitioners

- Despite a belief that it would be difficult to attract men to health services, they proved to be keen to make and keep appointments at the targeted *Open for Men* clinic.

- Although men generally present with physical symptoms, once assured of time and confidentiality, more personal and emotional issues are often disclosed.

- Men need longer consultation times than women because of their difficulties in communicating.

Practical pointers

- A needs assessment exercise and staff training in advance of launching a service are very important.

- Staff at men's clinics need not all be men, but it is very important that male staff are always available.

- Publicity should be very carefully planned to reach a wide range of men, not just in medical settings.

References

Birth Control Trust & Family Planning Association 1984 Men, Sex and Contraception. Birth Control Trust, London

Calman K 1993 On the state of the public health for the year 1992. HMSO, London

NHS Centre for Reviews and Dissemination 1997 Effectiveness matters. Screening for prostate cancer. NHS Centre for Reviews and Dissemination, York

Pownall M 1985 Coaxing men back into the clinic. Health and Social Services Journal 95 (4977):1541

Ramsay L E, Haq I U, Jackson P R, Yeo W W 1996 The Sheffield table for primary prevention of coronary heart disease: corrected. Lancet 348:1251–1252

Stevens A 1987 Dying before our time. Lewisham and North Southwark Health Authority, London

Watson C 1989 Developing a 'well woman' service staffed by family planning-trained clerks, nurses and doctors. British Journal of Family Planning 5:53–61

16

Addressing skin cancer prevention with outdoor workers

Maya Twardzicki and Terri Roche

This chapter covers:

- outline of the project
- health promotion principles
- how the project was set up
- structure of the project
- evaluation of the results
- addressing a male audience
- barriers to overcome
- what worked well
- resource pack
- the way ahead
- key issues for practitioners
- practical pointers.

Introduction

Evidence shows there is a need to target men with health promotion as they generally use health services less frequently than women (ONS 1996). A Mori poll found that 46% of men felt they did not know where to find health information (Caroll 1994). This indicates that health settings may not be the most appropriate way of reaching men, and alternative ways need to be considered. We explored the feasibility and effectiveness of workplace health promotion.

The opportunity to do this came in a nationally and locally identified need for a strategic approach to skin cancer prevention.

Skin cancer is the second most common cancer in the UK (Health Education Authority 1998) and registration rates in East Surrey are significantly higher than the national average (Public Health Common Data Set 1995). Yet this disease is largely preventable by minimising exposure to, and protecting the skin in, the sun. A key target group were outdoor workers, who are at risk of skin cancer because they spend extended periods of time in the sun. They are a predominantly male population, often mobile and from social classes IV and V, and can be considered particularly hard to reach with health messages.

Outline of the project

The aims of the project were:

- To adopt a participatory approach to influencing outdoor workers' attitudes, knowledge and behaviour regarding sun safety.

- To ensure sustainability of the project, exploring and negotiating with staff and management effective and feasible sun safety measures to implement at work.

Central to the project were:

- Recognition of the joint responsibility of individuals and the organisation for implementing sun safety at work.

- Client participation in the workshops to both address the problem of maintaining men's attention (management expressed concern about this), and discuss the feasibility of sun protection methods at work.

Health promotion principles

As this was a pilot project we found little evidence of effectiveness to draw on. It was therefore important to evaluate this approach to workplace health promotion, which was new to the employers, staff and ourselves. To help secure funding, it was also important to demonstrate that the project was built on sound health promotion principles and drew on relevant theoretical approaches, some of which are outlined below.

Adult learning theory and empowerment

Clients are valued as equals who have knowledge, skills and experience to contribute (Ewles & Simnett 1999). This represents a shift away from the traditional expert-led approach to a more bottom up approach. Men's participation in the workshop was vital and we emphasised the importance of their knowledge and opinions in shaping its outcomes. We explained to the men that they were experts who could identify how feasible sun safety measures were for their work circumstances, or how they may need to be adapted.

Educational approach

In this approach, knowledge and information are provided, and help is given so people can develop the necessary skills to be able to make informed choices about their health behaviour (Naidoo & Wills 2000).

Social change approach

The focus is at the policy level, to bring about changes in the physical/social/economic environment to promote health (Ewles & Simnett 1999). For example, sunscreen is an available but expensive healthy choice. To make it a more realistic option for outdoor workers, we negotiated provision of cheaper bulk-sized sunscreen with a supplier.

Reflective practice

This was employed after each workshop and management meeting, to develop and improve the work (Schon 1987). This uses experimential learning summarised in the model: do, review, learn and apply (Dennison & Kirk 1990).

Evaluation

Good practice was followed by planning the evaluation from the outset (Funnell, Oldfield & Speller 1995) so that it was integral to the project. The evaluation used both process and outcome measures.

Information and learning theory

These were drawn on to make the format and content of the workshops relevant to the target audience, so that learning was more likely to occur (Daines, Daines & Graham 1990). To cater for the great range in literacy levels and lack of experience of attending training, the workshops:

- used a lot of visual methods to present information
- were participatory in nature
- were limited to 1–1.5 hours to help maintain audience interest.

Using a combination of methods also helps increase the amount remembered – Dale's Cone of Experience (Wiman & Meierhenry 1969).

How the project was set up

We contacted local employers of outdoor workers and arranged meetings with enthusiastic key players to outline the rationale and benefits of the project. We had to appreciate that health promotion was not initially high on their priority list (as other safety issues posed more immediate threats than long-term risks of skin cancer), but perseverance and making arrangements as convenient as possible for employers paid off and we succeeded in securing both statutory and private sector participation.

Key to securing employer participation was making project arrangements client centred and flexible, given the financial and contractual implications of releasing staff for training during work hours. Client-centred arrangements included:

- conducting workshops on their premises and at times identified by employers as convenient
- incorporating additions to the draft programme suggested by managers (e.g. on heatstroke).

Managers of a construction company on the M25 were pleasantly surprised that we could conduct workshops before the start of their 7 am shift, thereby saving them time and the expense of transporting staff back to base from a site.

Structure of the project

The project was made up of three parts:

1. an initial participatory workshop
2. a follow-up workshop
3. a meeting with management.

The aims of the initial participatory workshop were:

- to explore the men's attitudes, knowledge and behaviour regarding tanning and sun safety
- to provide information about the risks of solar radiation and skin cancer and effective protection measures.
- to explore the feasibility of sun protection at work
- to provide information about early detection of skin cancer.

The aims of the follow-up workshop were:

- to evaluate the men's knowledge and practice of sun safety behaviours since the last workshop
- to explore how implementing sun safety at work could be made more feasible
- to answer any questions
- to explore men's opinions about the most appropriate ways to reach them with health promotion.

The aim of the management meeting was to negotiate sustainable sun safety measures within the organisation.

Evaluation of the results

Some of the evaluation and outcome data from all three parts of the project are described here, starting with workers' views about the initial workshop.

This session was useful because:

- 68% 'it made me more aware of the dangers of sun exposure.'
- 35% 'it informed me about how to protect my skin.'
- 5% 'it answered my questions.'

There was a general attitude change towards considering a tan to be more unhealthy after the workshop.

When I go back to work I will:

- 69% 'protect myself better in the sun.'
- 14% 'be more aware of the dangers of the sun.'

Follow-up workshops showed some workers had adopted these changes at work and in their spare time. Evaluation of the sessions revealed the following views.

If I'd been running the session I'd have:

- 63% 'not made any changes. I was quite happy with it.'
- 7% 'shown photographs of younger skin cancer cases and used more shock tactics.'

These changes were incorporated into subsequent workshops.

The organisational sun safety outcomes agreed at management meetings included:

- the provision of free and subsidised sunscreen for outdoor workers
- staff uniforms changed to offer more protection (e.g. legionnaires' hats and collared shirts)
- sun safety written into their Health & Safety manuals and talks
- a recommendation that similar sun safety workshops be conducted with all company staff.

Addressing a male audience

We found that being female trainers from an outside organisation gave us a novelty value in an almost exclusively male environment. This worked to our advantage for gaining men's attention before starting the workshops. We also found that the often large groups of men self-regulated their potentially disruptive banter more with two female trainers. This was done with comments such as 'Stop messing around: I want to hear this' (from a construction worker), or with humour.

We were aware that such groups were not a forgiving audience and managers had been concerned about this, offering to sit in to 'control' the men. After one such session the construction manager commented: 'Normally it's hard to keep their attention for 15 minutes and you managed it for an hour and a quarter ... I initially sat in because I was concerned that they would play up, but it soon became apparent I wouldn't be needed'. In organisations with a strong 'them and us' culture between management and staff, we felt it worth the risk to not have management present, in the hope that the workers would feel less inhibited and participate more.

We found it useful to play along with and capitalise on the strengths of the men's humorous banter, as humour is an effective way of getting a message across. For example, although we used a few stereotypical cartoons that some professionals may not consider politically correct, the evaluations showed they had the beneficial effect of getting the message across about different sites for skin cancer on men and women. Engaging with their lively sense of humour made the workshops a refreshing and enjoyable experience for us.

The men seemed more comfortable jokingly disclosing information about each other rather than about themselves – for example, regarding their experience of sunburn. We also found they were more forthcoming after we disclosed some personal experience of sunburn, thereby acknowledging the difficulty of trying never to get caught out in the sun, and showing we were not paragons of virtue. Despite the fact that shock tactics are generally not favoured by health promotion, evaluation showed the men found them effective, as they helped the long-term risk of skin cancer become more real in an environment posing many immediate risks to their health and safety. For example, everyone wanted to see the photographs of skin cancer that we had left as optional, and they even suggested we add some more gory ones. Men also suggested it would have greater impact on them to speak bluntly about skin cancer rather than using softer terms like skin damage.

We considered how we should dress for these workshops, given the combination of our all-male target group and the construction site environment. We felt it was appropriate neither to dress too femininely nor to power dress, but rather to wear practical trousers and flat shoes.

Barriers to overcome

We were frequently faced with less than ideal training venues due to the physical constraints of some of the workplaces. For example, in Portakabins on the edge of motorways, electricity supply fluctuated unpredictably, and we had to accept and work around the difficulties by using a flip chart instead of an overhead projector. It was not always possible for us to arrange the room in an informal layout that would facilitate participation. We found that where men could 'hide behind' desks, this had a negative effect on their behaviour, with some men jokingly acting as they would in school by putting their hands up to ask questions and making 'Please Miss, can I ...' comments. Where we could not alter the room layout, it helped if we sat down too and the joking then tended to die down as the workshop got underway.

There were several differences between us and our audience in terms of gender, age, social class and geographical origins, which could potentially have made us less acceptable to them. It helped that we had some previous experience of working with similar groups, which ensured our workshops moved away from the expert-led approach to a more participatory one. This was more empowering for the men and meant that sun safety messages were not preached from an ivory tower, but their feasibility discussed in the light of constraints inherent in their jobs and work environments.

Some groups tended to place responsibility for sun safety solely with management and to help overcome this potential barrier, we included a participatory brainstorming about sun safety measures, with separate action columns for individuals and management.

What worked well

This work was challenging because male outdoor workers were a new target group for us, and health promotion was new to the men and their organisations. Neither we nor the management were sure how the initiative would be received. We were all pleasantly surprised by the successful outcomes of the project and the positive evaluations from the men. As one construction manager commented: 'It is not easy to keep the attention of workmen for $1\frac{1}{2}$ hours and they managed ... the format is perfect'. Overall we found the whole experience thoroughly enjoyable and learnt a lot in the process. It was satisfying to work directly with the client group (rather than via other professionals), where we could see that our work had a direct impact on the men's attitudes, knowledge and behaviour regarding sun safety.

It was very important to find out about men's attitudes and knowledge regarding sun safety prior to setting up the project, so that we could start from where they were at and remain within the limits of their acceptance. These are key factors when trying to change attitudes (Egger, Donovan & Spark

1993). For example, if workers were very keen on having a tan, we focused more on avoiding sunburn rather than avoiding a tan completely, as this could have led to resistance.

We also felt it important to find out about the nature of each group of outdoor workers, their jobs and literacy levels, so we could pitch our language appropriately. Given the different educational levels among this target group, we needed to avoid baffling them with overcomplicated terms, or patronising them with oversimplified language.

Incorporating plenty of participation from the men was key to the success of the workshops. For example, in factual sections we first asked the men what they knew and then filled in their gaps with information. This was also more empowering for the men, and we found that many had some knowledge of sun safety learnt from popular media such as morning television.

Workers told us they appreciated being asked for their input and opinions, as it seemed this rarely, if ever, happened otherwise. They gave constructive feedback, having been told their knowledge and experience were integral to the success of implementing feasible sun safety measures, and that their suggestions would be fed back anonymously to management by independent facilitators.

Consultation and negotiation at both worker and management level meant that the sun safety recommendations developed were both realistic and specific to the needs of each organisation. These client-centred recommendations were more likely to be implemented by management and accepted by the workers.

We found co-training useful for:

- providing support in a sometimes challenging environment, particularly with large groups
- having one person to facilitate and another to take notes of participants' comments and pick up on any points the facilitator may miss
- reflective practice.

Making reflective practice an inherent part of our work provided us with the benefits of objectivity and hindsight, which were key to the continual development and improvement of the project. Although it may seem difficult to find time to review what went well and less well in a workshop/meeting, we found that doing this and applying the learning from it is time usefully spent.

Resource pack

Since skin cancer resources specifically for outdoor workers are scarce and our sustainable intervention had been evaluated as successful, we felt that writing it up into a resource pack could share good practice with other professionals, save them time and effort and hopefully increase skin cancer prevention work for this target group around the UK. We worked with the Health Education Authority to nationally pilot, evaluate, publish and distribute the pack, called *Addressing sun safety with outdoor workers: a workplace intervention pack*. It is a comprehensive resource containing guidance, training materials and background information, which can be used either 'off the shelf' or adapted to suit particular needs. (For more details about the pack, see Appendix 1.)

The way ahead

Our evaluation showed that 100% of the workers considered the workplace an appropriate setting in which to address health issues with men. They also felt participatory workshops were the most suitable means of delivering and sharing information. We plan, therefore to use a similar methodology to address other health issues with 'hard to reach' male populations.

Key issues for practitioners

- Evaluation and a sound theoretical base were important in justifying this health promotion work to employers and funders.
- It was important to assess men's attitudes to sun safety prior to the workshops, so that they would start within the limits of their acceptance.
- Men appreciated the participatory style and being asked their opinions.
- Consultation with management as well as with workers meant that sun safety recommendations were more likely to be implemented and accepted.

> ## Practical pointers
>
> - A sense of humour helped to get the message across.
> - Being women workers in an all-male working environment was useful in regulating distracting banter.
> - Shock tactics (e.g. pictures of skin cancers) were found by the men to be effective and realistic.

References

Caroll S 1994 The Which? guide to men's health. Consumers' Association, London

Daines J, Daines C, Graham B 1990 Adult learning, adult teaching. University of Nottingham, Nottingham

Dennison B, Kirk R 1990 Do, review, learn, apply. Blackwell, Oxford

Egger G, Donovan R, Spark R 1993 Health and the media. McGraw-Hill, Roseville, NSW

Ewles L, Simnett I 1999 Promoting health – a practical guide. 4th edn. Baillière Tindall, Edinburgh

Funnell R, Oldfield K, Speller V 1995 Towards healthier alliances. Health Education Authority, London

Health Education Authority 1998 Skin cancer: the facts. Health Education Authority, London

Naidoo J, Wills J 2000 Health promotion – foundations for practice. 2nd edn. Baillière Tindall, Edinburgh

ONS 1996 General Household Survey. HMSO, London

Public Health Common Data Set 1995 Department of Health, London

Schon D 1987 Educating the reflective practitioner. Jossey-Bass, San Francisco

Wiman R V, Meierhenry W C (eds) 1969 Educational media: theory into practice. Merril, Colombus, Ohio

17

Healthcare for male prisoners

Christina Evans

Introduction

The 65 600 prisoners in England and Wales are mostly young, male and from our inner cities. Ethnic minorities and the partly skilled are over-represented (Howard 1994, White, Cullen & Minchin 1999). Although the prison population is only 0.1% of the nation, the turnover of prisoners is high: in 1999 there were over 200 000 new receptions.

Many prisoners bring with them the baggage of failed healthcare and education, and a social system which has allowed them to become physically or mentally damaged. Many have drug and substance abuse problems and serious communicable diseases (Caton 1998). All of these people will come into contact with a prison doctor during their time in custody, and this can offer prisoners the opportunity for consistent healthcare, which may well have been absent from their lives outside prison. This puts pressure on the prison healthcare services to detect, diagnose and treat illnesses and disease in new arrivals. Additionally, the service must also care for those who fall ill whilst in custody.

Masculinity and conditioning

Daily life inside prison is tough. Men live among volatile, potentially violent and frustrated peers. To conform to an acceptable code of conduct, men must be self-contained, 'hard' and seen not to comply with the prison administration. An outward appearance of being able to protect themselves is essential. Confrontations frequently result in violence amongst inmates and cost them remission and privileges.

Inmates seemingly unable to cope will inevitably be picked on and may become victims of brutality. Such men, once identified, are housed separately and given work and recreation programmes apart from the rest of the gaol. They are despised by other prisoners, both for their weakness and the special treatment they are afforded. They are generally assumed to be sex offenders (nonces) by their peers.

In custody it is easy for the inmate to become withdrawn and not seek help for his problems. Alternatively, he may focus on health or relationship problems, and their significance may become heightened.

Coping with relationships is difficult in prison: visits are restricted, letters take time, possibly being intercepted, phone calls are limited for financial reasons, and there are sexual frustrations. As a result, partnerships often falter at a time when the prisoner is most vulnerable and needs moral support.

Drug-dependent prisoners may find daily life difficult, especially if they do not seek help and instead attempt to continue their habit. The perceived effect of drugs is heightened in prisons: men say they get an extra 'buzz', because they are kicking against the system.

Lack of privacy on the wings and also during visits can also contribute to an inmate feeling unwilling or unable to discuss private matters.

Male prisoners seem to have a poorer understanding of health issues than female inmates, who are generally well informed. Men tend to be unsure how their bodies work. Many have theoretical knowledge of, for example, safe sex, but they do not always put this into practice. Sometimes prisoners are unaware that they are ill and need treatment.

Physical health

Prisoners have long been shown to be disadvantaged in terms of social background and health status (Smith 1984, Smith 1992, Walmsley, Howard & White 1992). Prisoners are generally less healthy than Occupational Class V and smoking is more common than in the general population (Chambers, Evans & Lucking 1995). Physical injuries resulting from fights are common in custody, and are one of the main reasons prisoners attend Healthcare Centres.

Mental health

Many prisoners have mental health problems (Birmingham, Mason & Grubin 1996, Brook et al 1996, Singleton et al 1998). This may be due in part to the fact that the mentally ill are mistakenly placed in prison. A snapshot taken in 1996 by the Prison Service indicated that 3.8% of the prison population had some degree of mental disorder requiring intervention such as transfer to a psychiatric hospital or inpatient treatment in a prison Healthcare Centre (Longfield 1996). Brooke et al (1996) found that over half of remand prisoners need similar help.

Suicide and self-harm

The suicide rate amongst prisoners is several times that of their peer group in the community, and during the period 1972–87 had been rising disproportionately faster than the prison population (Dooley 1990). In 1996 the number of suicides in custody was 64; this rose to 82 in 1998. Dooley found that the prison situation and mental disorder accounted for about half of suicides. Subsequent research programmes have shown that prison regimes and staff responses influence suicidal behaviour (Ramsbotham 1999).

A disproportionate number of the suicides occur in men on remand who belong to several high risk groups: Maden et al (1995) found that:

- 13% had a history of psychiatric inpatient treatment
- 30% had had one or more episodes of deliberate self-harm (this figure rose to 40% among young offenders)
- 40% had a history of substance misuse
- 70% were unemployed (80% of young offenders).

Identification of potentially suicidal prisoners has proved difficult. In Dooley's study, over 50% of suicides had been seen by a doctor in the week before their death; in just 16% was the risk noted and acted on (Dooley 1990). In 1996 the Directorate of Health Care accepted that only a very small number of those who died had been officially deemed to be sucidial. All prison staff receive training in suicide awareness, but this has not stemmed the increase in suicides.

Even allowing for the increase in the prison population, the trend for self-harm has been growing: from 1994/95 to 1995/96 there was a 26% rise. Research is needed to identify:

- the characteristics of those who harm themselves
- the reasons for the increase
- the best management practice (Longfield 1996).

Drugs

Drug abuse affects the health of many who are in custody (Brook et al 1996, Bellis et al 1997). Since the early 1990s there has been a dramatic increase in the use of illicit drugs, resulting in a disproportionate increase in the number of prisoners who are notifiable drug addicts (Joyce 1996). Home Office figures show an increase from 3057 in 1991/92 to 10 438 in 1995/96.

Mason, Birmingham & Grubin (1997) reported on the prevalence of drug and alcohol use and the extent to which prison reception screening detects this. The problem is consistently underestimated, with only around half the drug users and two-thirds of the problem drinkers being spotted. In addition, the quantities and numbers of different substances are also underestimated. The management of inmates with dependency problems can be poor and the provision of detoxification programmes is unusual.

Prisoners are unlikely to seek help with an addiction, perceiving that admitting such an illegal activity may incur further punishment. Some addicts express no desire to alter their lifestyles, affirming their intention to resume their habit on release.

Improved training in the management of drug and alcohol misuse for prison doctors has also been suggested (Wool 1997). Currently in prisons, a multidisciplinary approach to drugs and substance abuse is employed which is undergoing evaluation and expertise is constantly building (Caton 1998).

Mandatory drug testing (MDT) is a security measure which does not directly involve health care staff. Concerns that MDT may encourage a switch from drugs such as cannabis to those with a shorter metabolic persistence (e.g. heroin), have been noted. MDT does not operate at weekends in England and Wales, which means addicts can organise their injecting to reduce the chance of detection (Bird et al 1997).

The Scottish Prison Service, unlike that in England and Wales, provides sterilising tablets in accordance with the World Health Organisation's recommendations for the cleaning of injecting equipment (World Health Organisation 1993). Bird et al also recommend vaccination against hepatitis B for all prisoners, having found high rates of clinical infection amongst injecting addicts. Their low awareness of the risks generally exacerbates the problem.

HIV and AIDS

Little information is available on the prevalence of HIV in prisons (Bellis et al 1997). Data from 1995/96 suggested 0.2% of inmates were HIV-positive (Longfield 1996).

Overall, imprisonment has been found to reduce the incidence of injecting, but for those who continue, the levels of risk of HIV-infection and other problems are increased. Inevitably, exchange of subjects between prison and the general community means that the problem of HIV and AIDS in custody cannot be viewed in isolation (Bellis et al 1997). There is limited provision for counselling and help for AIDS- and HIV-infected inmates (Caton 1998).

The prison health care service

The planning and delivery of healthcare for prisoners in England and Wales, formerly the responsibility of the Prison Service, is now the joint responsibility of the Prison Service and the Department of Health. A new joint Prison Health Policy Unit and Task Force have been set up to ensure that staff from the Prison Service and the National Health Service cooperate to provide prisoners with access to healthcare that is equivalent to that available in the community.

Prison Governors remain responsible for the provision of healthcare and health promotion within each prison. This involves many staff other than the healthcare staff, but local Health Authorities now have a duty to assist and to include prisons in their planning. The changes are expected to bring improvements, particularly in access to mental health services for prisoners.

Staffing

The quality of care delivered to prisoners varies greatly. While some establishments provide a very good service, in many, healthcare is of a low standard. Some doctors are not adequately trained for the work they face, care sometimes fails to meet ethical standards and little professional support is available (Reed & Lyne 1997, Joint Prison Service & NHS Executive Working Group 1999).

Healthcare facilities vary widely too. Larger prisons employ a full-time doctor as Senior Medical Officer (SMO); smaller establishments have part-time or visiting doctors, usually local general practitioners. Doctors are supported by Health Care Officers (HCOs) who have various levels of experience and training, and sometimes, by trained nurses. Only 225 doctors work in prisons in England and Wales, 133 of whom are full-time and 92 part-time (Longfield 1999).

The HCOs or nurses are responsible for the day-to-day running of the Healthcare Centres. There may be a dentist, psychiatrist or other professional who also visits regularly.

Where necessary, prisoners are referred to 'outside' hospitals. Counselling is available through the chaplaincy and the Samaritans, who also train inmate 'Listeners'.

Health screening

Prison rules require all inmates to undergo health screening on admission, and to see a doctor within 24 hours of arrival. Reed & Lyne's research (1997) revealed that 86% of prisoners reported having had such an assessment. In some of the prisons they studied, inmates felt that they could not talk freely to medical staff, and they rated the quality of the healthcare as poor.

Prisoners generally are reluctant to discuss private and personal matters with prison staff – male prisoners being particularly reticent. Even healthcare staff are viewed with hostility. Our experience indicates a preference on the part of prisoners to withhold details, the prison's interventions being perceived as detrimental, intrusive and ineffective. This creates a barrier, rather than highlighting any pre-existing medical condition or health concerns. As a consequence, health problems may not be detected until they become more serious, and the inmate will have suffered needlessly. Later interventions may be more costly to both the prisoner and the healthcare team.

Reporting sick

Overall, 10% of prisoners report sick and are dealt with each day. In 1995/96, each inmate attended the Healthcare Centre an average of 35 times, since prisoners must visit the medical centre for all their needs, however minor.

Inmates, particularly young offenders (YOs), can be confused about the identity of medical staff. A study by Chambers, Evans & Lucking (1995) showed that male HCOs wearing white coats were sometimes mistaken for the doctor; conversely, HCOs wearing officer uniform were often viewed with suspicion.

No inmate may see the doctor alone – an HCO will always be present for protection purposes. In some establishments in the study over 50% of prisoners expressed confidentiality concerns. However, some younger male inmates welcomed the presence of HCOs to act as 'interpreters' during and after the consultation.

The percentage of inmates believing their medical histories to be confidential varied from 27% to nearly 70%, depending on the prison. Although medical details are confidential, different types of clinic held on set days make it difficult for an inmate to keep the nature of his visit private. Male prisoners may be particularly uncomfortable if they have an appointment to see the psychiatrist. Their peers may see them as individuals to be targeted for abuse and violence.

The study also revealed that consultations with doctors were perceived to be far less satisfactory then those with HCOs: 20–70% of inmates claimed their consultations with doctors felt rushed.

Barriers to good health

The main barriers to good health for men in prison are summarised below.

- Poor compliance, occurring when doctors' instructions are not followed because they are not understood or are believed to be inappropriate.

- Delivering healthcare whilst maintaining security and control of the patient and the safety of carers. Young male remand prisoners may be particularly difficult to treat effectively, as they can be extremely volatile and uncooperative.

- The perception, by male prisoners in particular, that the prison healthcare system is inferior, which stems from their deep hatred of the prison system.

- Variation in the quality of care between prisons, and variation in prescribing between prisons. Male inmates do not cope very well when the care they receive changes on transfer to another prison and this can add to their stress levels.

- Pre-existing medical conditions which may not be detected.

- Incarceration can heighten preoccupations with perceived problems. Because men tend not to confide in their peers, they may dwell on health problems far more than their female counterparts.

- A lack of awareness about health issues, by comparison with female prisoners.
- A perceived lack of privacy and confidentiality, due to the prison setting.
- Little control over diet. Inmates' stories about prison food are legendary! Whatever the true situation, poor presentation, lack of choice and budget limitations are issues.
- Poor communication skills during consultations. This may be due to prejudice on both sides, or to class and cultural differences as well as the inmate's discomfort when talking about his health.

Good practice

Some examples of access to good health in prisons are listed below:

- Well Person and Lifestyle Clinics run by Care Teams to promote inmate health awareness.
- Annual Health Fairs bringing in outside agencies (including alternative therapists) to promote health issues. Male prisoners usually find such functions informative and entertaining, but their true value has yet to be assessed.
- Smoking information is available from some prison Healthcare Centres, but treatment such as nicotine patches is open to abuse and is seldom used.
- Education programmes address a variety of health subjects and are well received, being delivered by civilians who are better tolerated than uniform staff.
- Access to a gym and advice from PE staff on fitness and training are beneficial to mental health in a prison setting. Many male prisoners enjoy exercise, during which they can let off steam and make up for sedentary periods.
- Health promotion activities are run occasionally, but are limited by funding constraints.
- Free treatment and prescriptions.

The future

Health promotion

In conjunction with the World Health Organisation, the Prison Service launched a Health Promoting Prison Awards Scheme, encouraging individual prisons to adopt a multidisciplinary approach and develop projects promoting the health of prisoners, staff and visitors (Longfield 1996).

Health promotion 'inside' should focus on some specifically male issues, such as testicular cancer, as well as on more general topics. Activities must be presented in a way which is appealing to men, using language (even prison jargon) which will be easily understood.

Prisoners should understand that it is not a weakness to ask for help; rather that recognising and addressing a health issue demonstrates strength. Prisoners' general mistrust of the 'system' will not be eroded over night, but as improvements are made, confidence in the treatment received will increase.

The relationship prisoners have with healthcare staff is usually better than that with discipline officers. Nevertheless, adopting a multidisciplinary approach to some areas of health has already been successful and lessons could fruitfully be learned. For example, drug awareness courses run by discipline officers are attended as part of a prisoner's sentence plan. Frank evaluation (possibly through audit) is required to measure their true effectiveness.

World Health Organisation

The Prison Service for England and Wales has been designated a World Health Organisation collaborating centre for the European Health in Prisons Project. The aim of this is to exchange information on good practice and ultimately improve healthcare in prisons across Europe (World Health Organisation 1997).

Staff development

Recently, the special circumstances of the prison population and regime have been recognised, and a Diploma in Prison Medicine established. This is a first step towards recognising the special needs of prisoners (Longfield 1999). The course covers the following areas:

- psychiatry
- primary care
- genitourinary medicine and HIV
- audit
- management
- public health
- health and safety with occupational health
- information technology
- ethics and medicolegal aspects.

Health screening

Health screening in prisons is not always effective. In particular, there are probably many prisoners with some form of mental illness either undiagnosed, or misdiagnosed, who are therefore not receiving appropriate medical treatment. It has been shown that prison officers can help to recognise these inmates as they routinely observe behaviour as part of their duties (Birmingham 1999). The involvement of the WHO, coupled with the greater involvement of the NHS, should mean that screening becomes more effective for all types of health problems.

Healthcare provision

The 1999 NHS Executive report identified a range of actions to improve healthcare provision for prisoners. These are:

- The care of mentally ill prisoners should develop in line with NHS mental health policy and national service frameworks.

- There should be improved identification of mental health needs at reception screening.

- Mechanisms should be put in place to ensure the satisfactory functioning of a Care Programme Approach within prisons and to developing mental health outreach work on prison wings.

- Prisoners should receive the same level of community care within prison as they would in the wider community (Smith 1999).

Conclusion

Until recently, the delivery of healthcare to prisoners was the responsibility of the Prison Service, which has received much bad press over the years. However, it should be noted that in some establishments, the healthcare provided was of a good standard. The major argument in favour of the NHS running the Prison Health Care Service is that there should be consistent healthcare in all prisons, particularly for the mentally ill. Clearly, the NHS involvement should smooth the transition from community to custody and the health screening of new reception inmates.

However, the NHS is an institution with its own all too well documented problems. Furthermore, the methods of healthcare used by the NHS in the community may not be appropriate in prisons. Hopefully, the considerable expertise currently available in prisons will be put to good use in the future.

The improved health of our prisoners ultimately means a healthier community.

Key issues for practitioners

- Many prisoners arrive in prison in poor mental or physical health.

- The macho code of conduct amongst prisoners accentuates difficulties in dealing with health problems.

- Many health problems are exacerbated by the prison system, leading to high rates of mental health problems and suicide, and extensive drug abuse.

- Poor communication between prisoners and staff means health problems can go undetected.

- Prisoners' hostility to staff accentuates the difficulties.

Practical pointers

- Use of outside agencies gets a good response from prisoners.

- Addressing health problems in an education setting appeals to prisoners more.

- Fitness and exercise are good channels for male prisoners.

References

Bellis M A, Wield A R, Beeching N J, Mutton K J, Syed Q 1997 Prevalence of HIV and injecting drug use in men entering Liverpool prison. British Medical Journal 315:30–31

Bird A G, Gore S M, Hutchinson S J, Lewis S C, Cameron S, Burns S (on behalf of the European Commission Network on HIV infection and hepatitis in prison) 1997 Harm reduction measures and injecting inside prison versus mandatory drug testing: results of a cross-sectional anonymous questionnaire survey. British Medical Journal 315:21–24

Birmingham L 1999 Prison officers can recognise hidden psychiatric morbidity in prisoners. British Medical Journal 319:853

Birmingham L, Mason D, Grubin D 1996 Prevalence of mental disorder in remand prisoners: consecutive case study. British Medical Journal 313:1521–1524

Brooke D, Taylor C, Gunn J, Maden A 1996 Point prevalence of mental disorder in unconvicted male prisoners in England and Wales. British Medical Journal 313:1524–1527

Caton B 1998 Delivering health care to prisoners. Gatelodge (Prison Officers' Association Magazine) February:16

Chambers R, Evans C, Lucking A 1995 A pilot project to assess the feasibility of a Medical Audit Advisory Group facilitating the introduction of audit in local prisons. Final project report. Available from: Centre for Primary Health Care, Stoke Health Centre, Honeywall, Stoke-on-Trent, ST4 7JB

Dooley E 1990 Prison suicide in England and Wales, 1972–87. British Journal of Psychiatry 156:40–45

Howard L 1994 Where do prisoners come from? Home Office Research and Statistics Department. Research Bulletin, Special Edition:36

Joint Prison Service and National Health Service Executive Working Group 1999 The future organisation of prison health care. Department of Health, London

Joyce L 1996 Drug use in prison: the current picture. Prison Service Journal 107:16–23

Longfield M 1996 Report of the Directorate of Health Care for Prisoners 1995–1996. HM Prison Service, London

Longfield M 1999 Opportunities for doctors in the prison service. British Medical Journal 318:7178

Maden A, Taylor C J A, Brooke D, Gunn J 1995 Mental disorder in remand prisoners. Department of Forensic Psychiatry, Institute of Psychiatry, London

Mason D, Birmingham L, Grubin D 1997 Substance misuse in remand prisoners: a consecutive case study. British Medical Journal 315:18–21

Ramsbotham D 1999 Suicide is everyone's concern: a thematic review. HMSO, London

Reed J, Lyne M 1997 The quality of health care in prison: results of a year's programme of semistructured inspections. British Medical Journal 315:1420

Singleton N, Meltzer H, Gatward R, Coid J, Deasy D 1998 Psychiatric morbidity among prisoners in England and Wales. HMSO, London

Smith R 1984 Prison Health Care. British Medical Association, London

Smith R 1992 Prison medicine: beginning again (editorial). British Medical Journal 304:134–135

Smith R 1999 Prisoners: an end to second class health care? British Medical Journal 318:954–955

Walmsley R, Howard L, White S 1992 National prison survey 1991. Main findings. HMSO, London

White P, Cullen C, Minchin M 1999 Prison Population Brief: September. Home Office, London

Wool R 1997 Screening remand prisoners for drug misuse could be improved by training doctors better. British Medical Journal 315:1541–1542

World Health Organisation 1993 Global Programme on AIDS: WHO guidelines on HIV infection and AIDS in prisons. WHO, Geneva

World Health Organisation 1997 Health in prisons project. Directorate of Health Care, Home Office, London

18

Promoting black men's health

Mina J Bhavsar

Introduction

Men have silent voices when it comes to discussing their health – or at least this was the position stated by the Chief Medical Officer, Kenneth Calman, in his annual report for 1992 (Calman 1993). So to view men as a 'minority' when accessing health information would be apt.

Take this one step further and you have a group who are a minority within a minority: black men. (For the purposes of this chapter we will use the term black to include members of the Asian community – in particular those originating from the Indian subcontinent and East Africa – and the African-Caribbean community.) Indeed, Balarajan & Raleigh (1993) elaborate on the five key areas of the Government's White Paper *The health of the nation* (Department of Health 1992) and highlight coronary heart disease and mental health as being issues of particular concern to black groups.

A health and lifestyle survey of some 4000 members of black and minority ethnic groups commissioned by the Health

Education Authority (1994) found that health education messages were not penetrating the black community. The survey indicated an over-reliance on general practitioners for information. This is of concern when considering men, as research and news items indicate that men only tend to visit their GP as a last resort (see e.g. Cooper 1996).

Other research on minority ethnic groups has been predominantly disease-focused, and so to capture the complexities and structural inequalities underlying the foundation of the communities one has had to rely on local small-scale qualitative studies, usually conducted with limited resources.

Of concern also are the mortality differentials between migrants in the UK (Office of National Statistics 1997). Mortality rates for men of minority ethnic origins are disproportionately higher then those of the indigenous population. There are also differences between the migrant groups. For instance the overall mortality rate in Bangladeshi men is higher than that in Indian men. Men born in East Africa or the Indian subcontinent appear to suffer a higher number of deaths from ischaemic heart disease than men from the Caribbean. However, Caribbean men appear to suffer disproportionately from cerebrovascular diseases such as strokes. Not surprisingly lung cancer is highlighted as one of the major causes of death for all groups.

Reasons for these discrepancies are varied, but studies in America have begun to explore the correlation between stressors such as failed job prospects, and the social disadvantage experienced by these groups, to help explain the differences in mortality rates between whites and blacks (Kochanek et al 1994).

An element of understanding

Lefebvre (1991) described a health promoter as having three roles:

1. health educator
2. social marketer
3. politician.

An effective social marketer provides the template for problem-solving which interfaces with the theory and knowledge of the user. The marketer has to be appreciative of the social and cultural determinants of individuals' behaviour in order to develop effective health education material and also be in a position to enable, advocate and mediate as outlined in the Ottawa Charter proposed by the WHO (1986).

The structural pressures and oppression that men from black communities have had to and continue to endure, have a bearing on their health. Totmen's study (1979), indicated that certain stressors exacerbate illnesses. Although each stressor is unique to the person, both social and geographical mobility factors certainly play their part.

The second and third generation black males born in this country have in some way been cushioned by their forefathers from factors such as alienation. This has also had some bearing on the way black cultures have taken shape in the West. Migrating to new worlds for many minority ethnic men has in some sense meant a stronger need to hang on to their roots, to help maintain cultural identity.

There has been much media interest in the dual roles enacted by black youth, especially in terms of the west–east ideology. For many this is true. In the wider context where the man is very much exposed to the western lifestyle, peer and institutional pressures will be far different from his inner world, which may be encapsulated and heavily influenced by paternal and cultural values. The black man of today is still very driven by the ideology filtered down to him from his father or male role models when he was young. These have set precedence for what is deemed to be acceptable behaviour for a man, what his duty and role in society are. One Asian colleague summed it up by saying:

> Asian men for generations have always taken the front seat. In the sense of equality we are perhaps one step behind the western model, where there appear to be no real defined roles for men and women any more.

It is important to understand the origins of various demands on certain cultures which have left tremendous impressions on the lifestyle patterns of communities. For example, for African-Caribbean men, physical fitness is still high on the agenda. This is not necessarily due to vanity, but may originate from slavery where only the fittest survived.

It is also important to bear in mind that different cultures have different beliefs about medicine and health patterns. Meadows (1997) looked into reasons for the underutilisation of mental health services by the Asian community in America and found communities do not feel mainstream services cater for their beliefs. For example, in traditional Chinese culture many diseases are attributed to the imbalance of yin and yang, and the goal is to restore balance, through exercise and diet. In terms of health promotion it is important to design programmes which accommodate such beliefs. Otherwise, efforts may be wasted.

Black groups are often cautious about the motives and intentions of the establishment sending out health messages. If they are unable to identify with the source of information, then the message may well be ignored. Effective health promotion needs to come from recognised, trusted sources. The onus is on the health promoter to seek these out.

Health promotion

One question health promoters dread being asked is: 'what is health promotion?' Whatever way one views it, there really is no right or wrong answer. The *Official Journal of the European Communities* (Commission of the European Communities 1997) introduces the field as being concerned with healthy lifestyles and the creation of supporting environments. This involves intersectoral and multidisciplinary approaches in various settings. The notion encompasses health, public health, prevention and promotion of health spheres.

The keywords in this definition are *healthy lifestyles* and *multidisciplinary approaches*. Why? Because they are subject to interpretation.

Healthy lifestyles

A 'healthy' lifestyle depends on the standard of measurement against which the lifestyle is being assessed. Misinterpretations can easily lead to the development of victim blaming strategies. For example, in the 1970s and 80s campaigns such as *The Asian Mother and Baby Campaign*, *The Surma* (about the dangers of lead in eye cosmetics) and *The Stop Rickets Campaign* were accused of blaming the behavioural habits and lifestyles of groups without really trying to understand the socio-economic or environmental factors which may have initiated or exacerbated the issues.

By focusing on a deficit model of health and illness, one fails to understand the root problems that exist for black groups, or the obstacles they encounter such as racism, or structural disadvantages in accessing services.

If promoters do not comprehend the cultural and sociological values of a socially diverse population, they may end up viewing what are perceived to be the inferiorities or deficiencies of that group as being the determining health factors. Therefore, any practitioner contemplating health promotion work with black men must first reassess his or her own social standing and construction of knowledge, because they may be deeply rooted in western ideology, emphasising independence rather then interdependence. The practitioner must revisit, analyse and dissect his or her prejudices, stereotypes and pre-conceived expectations of the target audience. By taking this initial step the health promoter will stand some chance of success in working with marginalised groups.

Multidisciplinary approaches

It is not the meaning of the words 'multidisciplinary approaches' which is of interest here, but rather their application by practitioners working with black men. The ability to think laterally and develop work models outside the normal domain of health promotion is essential. The most common mistake made by practitioners is to assume that existing approaches developed in a Eurocentric framework are transferable to multicultural settings.

This is well illustrated by the following examples of health promotion work carried out in Leicester with men from minority ethnic groups.

Health promotion in Leicester

The Leicester census of 1991 showed that 28.8% of the population were from minority ethnic groups. In line with growing media and public interest in men's health, Leicester held a 1-day health conference in 1996, which attracted nearly 200 men from minority ethnic communities, including the Chinese, Polish and Ukrainian populations. The venue was a large modern community college located centrally, easily accessible by transport.

The conference proved to have various strengths and weaknesses. Some of the strengths were:

- A multiagency team was set up to coordinate the event. Representatives of various communities were invited to contribute, supported by both the Local and Health Authorities.

- An opportunity arose to work with other minority ethnic groups such as the Polish, Chinese, and Ukrainian communities, besides the African-Caribbean and Asian communities.

- Funding was available for the event.

- Interpreters were present for most languages.

- Qualified or experienced facilitators were invited to contribute.

- A variety of workshops were on offer to provide maximum choice.

- No real ceiling was placed on the age range of the target group.

- There was good media coverage about the day.

Some of the weaknesses identified were:

- The task group was led by a woman, and this was perceived as a threat by some male members.

- A large task group led to occasional conflicts about roles.

- There were too many workshops on different subjects, making allocation of interpreters very difficult.

- There was a very poor turnout of men aged 16–35.

- There was a very poor turnout of men from the African-Caribbean community.

- Holding the conference for a full day may have prevented some men, especially younger ones, from attending.

- There were limited amounts of translated material available.

- The majority of male facilitators were of South Indian origin, with the exception of one whose background was African-Caribbean. This did not reflect the ethnic mix of the participants.

Further evaluation of the event highlighted the following points:

- Minority ethnic men are a heterogenous group, with their own cultures and subcultures. The conference, although professing to be aimed at black men, failed to take into consideration the range of different cultural values, perceptions and needs, and so was not able to respond effectively to them.

- There were clear concerns about the lack of representation of men from the African-Caribbean community. This could have been because:

  - The African-Caribbean community may identify more readily with the term 'black' than 'minority ethnic groups'. Since the conference was promoted as an event for men from 'minority ethnic communities', African-Caribbean men may have felt excluded.
  - Not enough promotion took place in the right media and venues.
  - The men from this community may not have felt their needs or aspirations could have been properly serviced amongst such a diverse mix of participants.

- A lack of interpreters meant that some men were unable to attend the workshops of their choice. Also, a strong reluctance to attend a workshop on sexual health implied this subject was still taboo, even in all-male groups.

- The majority of men attending were over 50. Men below this age were not well represented. This may have been because the event was held on a Saturday, possibly conflicting with social activities, or because health is not given a high priority by younger men.

- Participants had mixed reactions to the conference. Those who had a personal interest in attending a particular workshop requested more of these events, whilst others felt that it was totally inappropriate to try to target a diverse male group. Some felt health grants should have been provided to community workers to enable them to work with men from their own community.

The lessons learnt from this experience are applicable to any practitioner proposing to work with men from black communities. To avoid repeating similar mistakes, a small qualitative study was conducted in Leicester, with a group of black men aged 22–45. The group had representation from the African-Caribbean and Asian communities. The aims were:

■ to explore the men's views and expectations of their roles in society
■ to gain a deeper understanding of their concerns and priorities about health and health promotion.

Although the results cannot be generalised, due to the small scale of the study, they are, nevertheless, intriguing:

■ All the participants were concerned about specific conditions currently in their family, such as diabetes and coronary heart disease, even though they did not appear to be suffering from them themselves. The African-Caribbean men were also concerned about hypertension and sickle cell anaemia (haemoglobinopathy condition).

■ A large majority saw their role as family breadwinners or potential breadwinners. They felt compelled to live up to this expectation imposed on them by their families and their respective social domains.

■ All interviewees said that it would take immense pain or suffering for them to go and see their family doctor. A majority resorted to going to the pharmacy instead. When asked how they viewed those men who made frequent visits to their GP, the answers varied from 'each to their own' to 'wimpish behaviour'.

■ Most indicated that they obtained their health information from their partners, mothers, or body building magazines (emphasis on the nutritional content). Some mentioned the church, radio and television.

■ Some felt that it was the expectation of society, and especially of women, that pressured men to maintain a 'macho' image, described by all to include a good 'physique'.

- Health was not really a high priority.

- Most indicated that they would not attend a health event, unless they had a specific reason for wanting to know about a certain condition.

- All stressed that they would probably not attend if sexual health was going to be the main topic covered.

- All said there were benefits in targeting black men separately from the indigenous population. They further stressed that black communities were not homogenous, and for effective health promotion work, practitioners needed to take this into account.

- A majority indicated that they would be receptive to health messages in the form of talks, leaflets etc. if they were delivered together with something else – for example in a gym or youth club, or at a sports event, bangra evening (Punjabi dancing), church or library.

- Most men said they would prefer a male practitioner, preferably of the same ethnic origin, to conduct health promotion work. They felt they would not be able to discuss issues such as prostate or testicular cancer with a female practitioner.

For health promotion practitioners the above are valuable indicators.

Conclusion

The issues raised in this chapter are by no means exhaustive. However, it is clear that all health promoters intending to work with black men need to be flexible enough to accommodate an understanding and acceptance of a world and life outside the western ideology, which is equally fitting and very much alive for groups they mean to serve.

Practitioners whose ethnic origin or language is not the same as the client group should not be deterred from working with such groups. On the contrary, they should view such work as a challenge, testing their own skills and determination to deliver effective health promotion to groups whose health is adversely affected by structural inequalities.

Practitioners must practise explicit reflexivity, which means they must assess their own social standing and construction of knowledge before embarking on any health promotion work. This will enable them to tease out any prejudices, stereotypes and myths embedded deep within them about the target group. They should also research as much as possible about the group they intend to work with.

Reaching minority ethnic men with health promotion messages is not easy. Practitioners need to be aware that minority ethnic communities are heterogenous in nature, and this must be reflected in the health promotion methods employed.

A certain amount of time will need to be devoted to preliminary, intermediary and post-project research. This may involve:

- Identifying key establishments and individuals who have already undertaken similar work around the country.
- Identifying key individuals and organisations in the community that you wish to work with, by contacting other colleagues, agencies, and groups.
- Making personal contact with the community and securing the respect and trust of the gatekeepers of the target population. This is by no means straightforward, but following strategies such as these will make it easier to access the male members of the community.
- Securing the services of appropriately trained interpreters well in advance of your activity. Ensure the interpreter speaks the correct dialect, especially when working with Bengali men.
- Listening to your target audience. Your intentions and priorities regarding health matters may not be the same as theirs, and you will have to respect this. You may have to employ unfamiliar methods in order to address the group's immediate concerns and incorporate your health message.

A committed health promoter who demonstrates a depth of understanding of other cultures, communities and groups will find success in promoting black men's health.

Acknowledgement

A personal thanks goes to those black men in Leicester whose invaluable contribution made this chapter possible.

Key issues for practitioners

■ Health education messages are not getting through to black men. In order to change this, practitioners need to develop an understanding of non-western ideologies.

■ The structural pressures on men from black communities continue to have a bearing on their health.

■ If health information comes from a source black men are unable to identify with, they will tend to ignore it.

Practical pointers

■ Practitioners should not be put off from working with men who are from a different ethnic group to themselves, or who speak a different language.

■ Time should be devoted to preliminary, intermediary and post-project research.

■ It is important to identify key individuals and organisations within the target community.

■ Interpreters should be used if necessary.

■ The target audience should be listened to.

References

Balarajan R, Raleigh V S 1993 Ethnicity and health: a guide for the NHS. Department of Health, London

Calman K 1993 On the state of the public health – 1992. HMSO, London

Cooper G 1996 So macho, but so many men fit for nothing. The Independent, 11 June

Department of Health 1992. The health of the nation. HMSO, London

Health Education Authority 1994 Black and minority ethnic groups in England: health and lifestyles. HEA, London

Kochanek K D, Jeffrey M A, Maurer M S, Rosenburg H M 1994. Why did black life expectancy decline from 1984 through 1989 in the United States? American Journal of Public Health 84(6):938–944

Lefebvre R C 1991 Promoting health promoters: professional development in health promotion. Health Promotion International 6:1–2

Meadows M 1997 Cultural considerations in treating Asians. USA Office of Minority Health Newsletter, September 1997

Office of National Statistics 1997 Health Inequalities. The Government Statistical Service, London

Work Programme 1997 of the Community Action Programme on Health Promotion, Information, Education, & Training. Official Journal of the European Communities 40 C18 (17 January)

Totmen R 1979 Social causes of illness. Souvenir Press, London

WHO 1986 Ottawa Charter for Health Promotion. Journal of Health Promotion 1:1–4

19

Sex education for young men

Mike Massaro

This chapter covers:

- why sexual health work with young men?
- sexual health issues relevant to young men
- the foreskin
- testicular self-examination
- relationships
- drugs
- exercises
- *The puberty game*
- *Anonymous questions*
- *Who's cool?*
- difficulties working with young men in schools
- evaluation
- key issues for practitioners
- practical pointers.

Introduction

The Health Opportunities Team is a community-based project which provides sexual health education to young people up to the age of 25 in Craigmillar, a medium-sized housing estate on the outskirts of Edinburgh with high rates of unemployment and social deprivation. The project acknowledges the importance of work with young men and for this reason has a male worker who focuses mainly on young men's sexual health.

Why sexual health work with young men?

Sex education is provided for young people as part of the school curriculum, but what is taught varies, depending on individual schools' policies and geographical location. In Scotland, The Education Act (1996) does not apply and there is no requirement to provide sex education, although guidelines were issued in 1994 by the Scottish Office which provide a framework for developing sex education programmes through primary and secondary schools. This in itself is an issue and explains why many schools do not dedicate a great amount of time to sex education.

Although sex education, when provided, is aimed at both boys and girls, it is rare for the focus to be on issues directly relevant to boys or young men. There are many reasons for this but in the main, the focus is on menstruation because it is an important aspect of puberty that girls need to learn about early on. With boys, however, the same sense of urgency does not apply and so in many cases boys' and young men's sexual health is forgotten.

Neglect of young men's sexual health has many implications in terms of physical health. These may include delayed noticing of testicular cancer, prostate problems or sexually transmitted infections – all of which could mean the difference between life and death, depending on how early or late treatment can be provided.

It is also important that emotional health be discussed in the proper context with young men. Many young men still grow up with the expectation that they will find a job, get married, have children and provide for their family. For many, however, this will not turn out to be the case, as they find that it is the female partner who is in employment. Men's role within relationships (and society as a whole) continues to change and it is therefore important that work is undertaken with young men that challenges the stereotypical male traits and roles so that they are not growing up with an expectation that is not real. Men who are not clear about their role in life can become frustrated, depressed or aggressive, and those closest to them, especially their partner, bear the brunt of this. Work must be undertaken, starting at an early age, looking at different roles, and especially around equality and respect within relationships, so that problems can be prevented rather than escalated.

Many valuable projects or organisations in this country have been set up focusing on the sexual health needs of young women. For this work to reach its full potential, it needs to be complemented by work with young men. For example, young women can be taught to be assertive in asking their partner to use a condom, but if the partner still refuses, then the end result may only be conflict. The ideal, therefore, is to work with young men as well as young women around the issue of condom use, so that both parties are approaching it from a similar perspective.

The main and most obvious reason for sex education to be directly targeted at young men, is the simple fact that there are so many issues related to men's sexual health – which men are often reluctant to discuss or know little about.

Sexual health issues relevant to young men

Many workers are unsure about what sexual health issues to address with young men. The main topics that we cover are:

- changes during puberty
- circumcision and foreskin
- condom use
- drugs and sex
- how to satisfy a partner
- hygiene
- impotence
- penis size
- pregnancy
- premature ejaculation
- problems with urinating
- prostate cancer
- relationships
- safer sex
- sexual activities
- sexual orientation
- STIs
- terminations.

Many of these topics, such as condom use, hygiene, pregnancy, relationships and safer sex should be covered with young women as well as young men. Unfortunately, when these topics are discussed in a mixed group, they tend to be very female-focused. This can lead to young men feeling that the subject matter is not relevant to them and so they switch off. If sexual health work is to be undertaken jointly with young women and young men, then it must be relevant to both sexes.

There is a general belief that young men are too immature to discuss sexual health issues in a productive way. This is another factor which results in young men not receiving the proper information that they require for later life. Although young men can be disruptive in sex education classes, this is often due to their embarrassment, as they are generally not encouraged to discuss sexual organs or their feelings towards other people, especially those they are attracted to. It is therefore vital that professionals get through the embarrassment stage with young men as this can, and does, lead to worthwhile discussions, some at a level the young men have never experienced before.

It is not possible here to examine all the sexual health topics in detail, but it is worth looking at some important points that are often neglected.

The foreskin

In a country where circumcision is not common practice, it is essential that young men are taught to pull back and wash behind the foreskin on a daily basis. If not, smegma can build up which if left, can result in infection. Boys sometimes complain that it is painful to pull back the foreskin over the head of the penis. If this is case, lathering soap and water with the hands and then pulling back can make it less painful. If the foreskin is very tight around the head of the penis then it may cause problems as it is possible for the foreskin to tear whilst having sexual intercourse. In such a case, it may be necessary for the young man to seek help from his GP.

It is also important that the foreskin can be pulled back for using condoms. If the foreskin is not pulled back then the condom is more likely to slip off during sexual intercourse.

Testicular self-examination

Testicular cancer is the most common cancer amongst men aged 16–25. It is therefore important that early on young men are encouraged and shown how to examine their testicles on a regular basis for abnormalities such as increased swelling or lumps forming on the testes. Considering the high success rate of treatment if caught early, it is vital that young men are taught how to undertake testicular self-examination.

Relationships

Relationships are a major area that we cover with young men, and in many ways can be much more difficult to tackle. Whilst other matters are mainly information based, this subject needs to be covered through discussion and attitude-based exercises. There is no definitive 'right' information about relationships to give to young men, but what we can provide is a forum where they can discuss concerns they may have and can be challenged about the traditional roles many of them believe in. We look at attitudes towards the opposite sex (as well as the same sex), equality, respect, honesty and negotiation – all of which contribute to the makings of a good, healthy relationship. It is important to remember to portray relationships in a nonbiased way, acknowledging that those we are working with are not all of the same sexual orientation, race, culture, class or religion.

Drugs

The young people we work with have more access to drugs than ever before. This being the case, it is important that sex is put in the context of drugs. Alcohol is a widely used legal substance taken before sexual activity and work needs to be undertaken with young men regarding the consequences of getting drunk before having sex. Various studies show that condom use is less likely if a couple are under the influence of alcohol and this may result in either unplanned pregnancy or sexually transmitted infections being passed on. Moreover, after having had several drinks, the likelihood of getting an erection is seriously reduced.

Recreational substances such as cannabis or amphetamines may also affect sexual activity for men. Cannabis, when taken in smaller doses can increase the sex drive but when taken in excess can reduce the ability to perform at all. Amphetamine sulphate, more commonly known as speed, generally results in men finding it difficult to get an erection. Once the penis is erect, however, men can generally perform sexually for much longer than usual before ejaculating. This again has implications for safer sex as condoms are more likely to be torn during vaginal or anal sex and damage is more likely to happen to the inside of the partner's vagina or rectum. It is therefore important that the condom is checked regularly for possible breakage.

Various drugs, whether they are stimulants or depressants, can affect sexual activity and it is important that men are made aware of the risks associated with using them.

Exercises

The bulk of our work with young men is undertaken in a local community high school. In our experience, these young men appreciate being in a single sex setting with us, as they tend to be more open and the discussion is much more productive. There are some exercises that we use very successfully, and although we mainly use them in schools they can be used in most settings.

The puberty game

The puberty game is taken from the Greater Glasgow Health Board pack *More Than A Game*. One participant is asked to draw around another on two pieces of flipchart paper stuck together length ways, and is then asked 'what changes happen to young men during puberty?' This exercise can generate much discussion and fun, especially when the young men have to draw the changes. As well as covering the physical and emotional changes, workers can also generate interest in such issues as hygiene procedures, testicular self-examination and circumcision. The puberty game is one of our most successful exercises for explaining sexual health matters to young men. Although we use it mainly with 10–12-year-olds we have also adapted it for use with older groups around the effects of drugs. For this we initially ask 'what effects do drugs have on the body?' and then focus on how drugs affect young men sexually.

Anonymous questions

This is an exercise that can be used with a range of age groups. Before going into a school or group it can be useful to ask for any questions that the group have regarding the subject matter. As well as using these questions to base the programme on, they can also be used as an exercise in their own right. The questions are typed up and put in a box, and participants are asked, one at a time, to pick out a question and read it to the group. It is made clear that it is the group's responsibility, not the individual's, to answer the question, so nobody is put on the spot. Once the question has been answered, the next participant pulls out a question. Workers can hold onto these questions after the session and use them with other similar groups in the future or if appropriate include questions of their own on specific subject matters. Having the questions typed means the group members will not recognise their peers' handwriting so the exercise is truly anonymous. It is successful because the questions are relevant to the participants and keep the group focused on a variety of subjects under the banner of sexual health.

Who's cool?

This exercise is aimed at 14–15-year-olds. We have developed it from other similar exercises that trainers use. In advance, cut out a selection of 20–30 pictures of men – famous actors, singers, comedians as well as other unknown men – from various magazines. Ensure there is a mixture of men of different sexual orientations and ethnic origins. Spread out the pictures and ask the group to put them into two piles: 'who is cool' and 'who isn't cool'. A debate is opened up to decide who falls into which category. As well as encouraging discussion around masculinity, appearance, attitude and career, this also facilitates discussion on sexual orientation. Having pictures of known gay or bisexual men who are either popular sportsmen or funny can be a good way of portraying that gay and bisexual men can be just as 'cool' as heterosexual men in society.

In our experience many exercises emphasise the discrimination that gay or bisexual men face. Although this is a fact of life and should be included in the discussion, we also have to acknowledge the impact of this type of discrimination on any young men in the group who may identify as gay or bisexual. This exercise can be led to look at various aspects of sexuality rather than solely focusing on the negative. Again, this exercise can be adapted to looking at issues around race, culture, disability or body image, depending on what the focus of the session is.

Although discussing sexual orientation has always been an aspect of our group work, the way in which we do it has changed. In the past we focused a session specifically on this issue, but these sessions tended not to work due to the abusiveness that came out during the discussion. The *Who's cool?* exercise covers a variety of topics, including sexual orientation and this, in our experience, is much more successful.

It is important to reinforce this exercise through the use of language. When discussing sex or relationships throughout the whole programme, it must not be assumed that the partner is necessarily of the opposite sex.

We use other successful exercises too, and what is generally most appreciated by the young men we work with is our attitude towards them as people. It is important to show them basic respect, to listen to what they are saying and, above all, not to judge them. Workers must also be enthusiastic, approachable, patient, like young men and enjoy being with them. This is the basis of all good practice and will make the use of exercises much more successful.

Difficulties working with young men in schools

One of the main difficulties working with young men in schools concerns confidentiality. Due to child protection guidelines young people under the age of 16 who disclose participation in any sexual activity have to be reported to the school. Although these guidelines are there to protect young people, many young men find this inhibiting and are more reluctant to talk openly. In our experience, young men trust the worker and therefore believe it is acceptable to disclose sexual activity that they are involved in. Even though the group are aware of the guidelines, they often believe the worker won't really inform the school. It is therefore important that workers stress what is acceptable and not acceptable whilst providing a forum for the group to speak as openly as possible. One way around this is to encourage participants to speak in the third person, so instead of discussing themselves, they discuss what their 'friend' is involved in. Workers, however, need to be constantly aware of possible disclosure and if necessary, prevent it through intervention if sensing a disclosure is about to take place. Workers also need to provide young men with information on services such as Brook Advisory Centres or specific youth services where they can be honest about nonabusive sexual activity without fear of confidentiality being broken.

Another difficulty which we constantly face whilst teaching sex education to young men is sexism and heterosexism. Many young men have strong negative feelings towards women and especially towards men who have sex with other men. If not dealt with sensitively by workers then sexist or heterosexist attitudes and feelings can be exacerbated. It is therefore essential that workers are clear about their position on these areas and have a clear idea of how they are going to challenge such discriminatory views.

Evaluation

Although all participants are asked to complete evaluation forms at the end of each training course, we often feel that these forms do not truly express the value of the sessions. In our experience, the young men evaluate the training on the basis of enjoyment and knowledge intake rather than on attitudinal change. Enjoyment is, with rare exceptions, rated highly whilst knowledge is rated in terms of increased learning – as many are reluctant to state that they did not know about the subject matter before the training. Participants do state that after training they have increased knowledge about changes to the body during puberty, STIs including HIV and AIDS, testicular self-examination and condom use. What we have observed is that the more work we undertake with a male group, the more sensible and productive the discussion usually becomes. Considering that the traditional perception of young men is that they are immature and disruptive when discussing sexual health, it is valuable to note that they can respond positively to issue-based work that is directly relevant to them.

Longer term benefits of sexual health education, such as reduction in teenage pregnancies, remain to be seen. In order to achieve a success in this area, sexual health training programmes require a higher priority in terms of Government funding, and single sex work with young men needs to be acknowledged as a vital complement to work with young women.

Conclusion

Our work in the local high school is continually being adapted and this contributes to the programme remaining fresh and exciting, for us and the pupils. The school staff have been extremely supportive and have encouraged us to develop our work in the school. Having felt that the initial mixed sex groups did not meet the needs of the young people we were working with, much more single sex work has been successfully introduced. The work with young men has developed further and spin-off groups have looked at various issues raised by participants themselves. These include young men and violence, and what it means to be a young man in today's society, which covers areas such as masculinity, relationships, power, aggression, emotional health, physical health and drug use.

Overall, working with young men has been an exciting aspect of the Health Opportunities Team's work and it is our intention that it will continue to develop over the coming years.

Key issues for practitioners

- Young men's sexual health has been neglected and this has implications for their physical health in terms of e.g. testicular cancer, prostate problems and STIs.
- Men's role in relationships is changing, so work on stereotypical male traits and roles is very important.
- Work with young men is needed to complement work done with young women, in areas such as promoting effective condom use.

Practical pointers

- Active and effective physical self-help care should be encouraged e.g. penile hygiene, testicular self-examination.
- Information-based work should not be focused on at the expense of relationship issues.
- Resource exercises such as *The puberty game, Anonymous questions* and *Who's cool?* can be highly successful.

20

Gay and bisexual men's general health

Graham Hart and Paul Flowers

This chapter covers:

- psychosocial health
- gay lifestyle and health behaviour
- the unconsidered health impacts of HIV/AIDS
- non-HIV sexual health
- gay men and health services
- key issues for practitioners
- practical pointers.

Introduction

There are both important similarities and important differences between homosexual (gay) and heterosexual (straight) men. Gay men are first and foremost of the male gender, and so they are subject to all the other health problems shared by men in general. Yet sexual behaviour sets them apart and it is therefore possible to be left with the impression that the 'only' health problem faced by gay men is sexual health. Since the early 1980s, gay men have been associated with one disease – immunodeficiency caused by HIV, resulting in AIDS. However, looking beyond sexual difference and shared physiological similarity, gay men, as opposed to other men, are vulnerable to unique health risks by virtue of the social context in which they live. Pervasive homophobia and heterosexism at the level of legislation, social policy and daily experience structure a set of inequalities which directly impact on health. A gay man is not only exposed to the same health risks as other men of the same social class, education, region of origin and ethnicity, but he has to contend with additional, gay-specific, health risks.

Because gay men have been defined medically in terms of what they do in bed rather than by other aspects of their lifestyles or health behaviours, they have been ill served by general health research; there is a plethora of studies on the sexual behaviour and sexual health of gay and bisexual men, but little on their risks of cancer, coronary heart disease or non-HIV psychiatric morbidity. It is therefore the case that much of what is written here must remain speculative, until we have a larger body of research to inform the broader health needs of gay and bisexual men. In this chapter, we present a variety of pertinent issues which relate to the health of gay men:

- psychosocial health
- health behaviours and the gay lifestyle
- the unconsidered health impacts of HIV/AIDS
- non-HIV sexual health and gay men
- health services.

The range of men who have sex with men is very wide. Here we focus on gay and bisexual men who use their local gay scene, and are more or less open about their sexuality to friends, family and workmates.

Psychosocial health

Although there are relatively few data on the psychosocial health of gay men, the existing literature does seem to suggest that gay men are particularly vulnerable to mental health problems. Until 1973 (when it was removed from the *Diagnostic and Statistical Manual*) homosexuality itself was considered to a be a psychopathology. Since the late 1970s several studies have charted the deleterious effects of heterosexism and homophobia on psychological wellbeing. Gay men appear to have significantly higher rates of psychological distress (Coyle 1993, Coyle & Daniels 1993) and attempted suicide (Jay & Young 1977, Gibson 1989) than heterosexual men. Erwin (1993) highlights the stress associated with the continuous nature of identity disclosure as gay men struggle to have both themselves and their significant relationships recognised. She goes on to list the probable negative consequences of discrimination in the workplace and in housing, coupled with a lack of role models, negative self-image, familial rejection and a fear of public identity disclosure. As the campaigning organisation Stonewall has demonstrated, large numbers of gay men have been subject to significant levels of violence (Mason & Palmer 1996). Victims of gay hate crimes have relatively elevated levels of depression and anxiety when compared to other gay men (Herek et al 1997). Similarly, Meyer (1995) shows that psychological distress in gay men could be predicted not only by actual events of discrimination and violence, but also by expected rejection, discrimination and internalised homophobia.

The relevance of many of these psychosocial issues will change across a given individual's lifetime. Vulnerability as well as protective mechanisms are likely to be associated with different temporal and social contexts. 'Coming out', for example, may be particularly stressful (Flowers et al 1998), whereas at other times gay men may be in a position to give or receive social support (Hart et al 1990). Though there is no research on this, it is also likely that gay men's health will in part be associated with their 'marital' or more correctly 'partner' status. Though there are clear differences between gay and straight relationships, it is probable, for example, that long-term relationships with male partners are protective for gay men's health in the same way as marriage or long-term cohabitation have been shown to be protective for heterosexual men, who experience less disease compared to single men (Macintyre 1992). In one study, Hart et al (1990) found that a third of gay men live alone. Gay relationships are less likely to involve cohabitation and are usually of shorter duration than their heterosexual counterparts (Kitzinger and Coyle 1995).

Gay lifestyle and health behaviour

The gay scene itself may contribute to ill health. The commercial gay scene in any large city comprises bars, clubs, gyms and saunas. Much of the socialising that is done takes place in bars and clubs, rather than contexts which are alcohol-free. Although there are many interest groups such as gay outdoor clubs, and gay-specific sports groups, most contact with other gay men is in a pub or club. There is in these situations every opportunity for alcohol abuse (see Bux, 1996 for a critical review). Whereas some heterosexual men who marry and have children have other demands on their income, gay men without family responsibilities have a larger disposable income, which may place them at increased risk of the deleterious and long-term effects of alcohol. The gay scene is also in great part youth-oriented, and a premium is put on physical good looks and attractiveness, which some men can find threatening or alienating (see Gold, 1995), and so the attractions of alcohol may again be heightened in these circumstances.

The emphasis on good looks and attractive physiques in the gay scene can have other, often unconsidered, consequences. Body image problems and eating disorders are reportedly more prevalent amongst gay men than straight men (Gettleman & Thompson 1993, French et al 1996). In metropolitan areas, particularly London, there is a category of gay men known by others as 'muscle Marys'. These are men who use gyms to weight train and increase body muscle. The illicit use of anabolic steroids to augment 'natural' body-building techniques has its own negative health sequelae, and when this is combined with injection and the sharing of injecting equipment, the consequences in terms of the transmission of blood-borne viruses can be severe.

If one's social life is to a large extent bar-based, then the opportunities for active and passive smoking are greater than in other circumstances. Gay men do appear to smoke more than their heterosexual counterparts (Skinner 1994). Bar staff in particular are exposed for long periods of time to smoke-filled atmospheres which, over a period of years, will undoubtedly increase their risk of the smoking-related diseases, even if they personally do not smoke. Anyone wishing to give up smoking would be well advised to avoid gay bars, as there is little incentive to desist from this activity in these contexts.

Recreational drug use is common among gay men. For example, in the USA Skinner (1994) found that gay men from metropolitan areas used marijuana more often than the general population (37.5% of gay men in the preceding month compared with 16.5% of men in general population surveys). Rotheram-Borus, Hunter & Rosario (1995) suggest that for gay youth, the use of drugs may be related to coping with societal stigma. However, certain gay clubs, like their heterosexual 'rave' counterparts, actually foster a culture of recreational drug use.

The prevalence of this type of drug use is unknown, but Ecstasy (MDMA), amphetamines, LSD and amyl nitrite are all associated with certain dance 'scenes'. Whilst for many, particularly younger gay men, such drug use is temporary and/or very occasional, the effects of longer term use are still not clear, and it remains to be seen what proportion of recreational users develop subsequent drug problems, including dependency.

The unconsidered health impacts of HIV/AIDS

It cannot be denied that the effect of HIV and AIDS on current generations of gay men has been massive and devastating. In the United States, AIDS is the major cause of mortality for all men in the age range 19–45. The majority of these men became infected through same-sex activity, although a significant proportion of HIV transmission in the States is related to drug injection and heterosexual intercourse. Rapid spread of HIV infection has been seen in virtually all large metropolitan gay communities in the developed world, with approximately 10% of gay men in London (Unlinked Anonymous Surveys Steering Group 1998), and as many as 60% of men tested in clinics in San Francisco and New York, being found to be HIV positive (Mann et al 1992).

The unconsidered impacts of HIV and AIDS affect not only those infected with HIV, but also those who have experience of it in others. In the late 1980s a study was conducted on a sample of over 500 gay men throughout England: 56% of the men recruited in London knew personally someone who had died of AIDS, and 29% – nearly a third – of London men had provided practical help and support to another gay man with AIDS (Hart et al 1990). These gross figures give some indication of the impact of the disease on the gay population, but behind them lie many individual stories of grief, heartache and often multiple loss, all of which have negative consequences for mental health (Nord 1996, Goodkin et al 1996).

Non-HIV sexual health

Sexual health for gay men has been dominated by AIDS. However, the increase in condom use to protect against HIV infection has actually produced other positive benefits. This was seen most markedly in the 1980s when there was a dramatic reduction in homosexually acquired syphilis and gonorrhoea (Johnson & Gill 1989), although since then there has been an increase in sexually transmitted diseases in gay men (Simms et al 1998). There are two sexually transmitted viral diseases that can be avoided by vaccination: hepatitis A and hepatitis B. Hepatitis A is usually associated with poor food hygiene, but can also be contracted as a result of sexual activity involving oral–anal contact (rimming). A single injection of vaccine, however, protects against this disease.

Hepatitis B is life-threatening, and is more infectious (and therefore more easily transmitted and contracted) than HIV. However, there is proven efficacy in preventing exposure to this disease through the administration of recombinant hepatitis B vaccine. The idea of making hepatitis B vaccine available on a universal, population basis, at birth has been debated, yet we are in a remarkable situation where those who are at most risk have yet to be offered the vaccine. Two studies, one in England in 1991–92 and the other in the west of Scotland in 1996, both found that only 44% of large samples of gay men had been vaccinated against hepatitis B (Hart et al 1993, Hart et al 1999).

Gay men and health services

Given the difficulties gay men face in many aspects of daily life it comes as no surprise that they face potential problems with access to healthcare services. A study of general practitioners in 1989 found that only 32.7% felt comfortable with gay men (Bhugra 1987). Similarly, 25% of members of a Canadian Medical School psychiatric faculty admitted they were prejudiced against lesbians and gay men (Chaimowitz 1991). In a survey of the American Gay and Lesbian Medical Association (Schatz & O'Hanlan 1994), 64% of respondents believed that patients had received substandard care as a result of sexual orientation disclosure to their physician.

In a UK study of 623 gay men registered with a general practitioner, 44% had not informed their GP that they were gay (Fitzpatrick et al 1994). And 44% of the 77 men who were aware that they were HIV antibody positive had not informed their GP that they were gay. Just under a fifth of respondents did not consider it important or relevant for their GP to know about their sexuality. Over 87% thought that GPs were an appropriate source of advice about HIV/AIDS, and 84% thought that they were an appropriate source of advice about safer sex for gay men. Yet this was in a context where 16% described their general practice as unsympathetic to gay men, and 22% reported that at some point they had experienced an inappropriate or insensitive comment from a GP about their sexual preference. Nineteen of these men described experiences such as receiving moralising lectures from their doctor about being gay. Although these situations probably constitute a minority of gay men's experiences of general practice, those men who had recently had any hospital treatment reported similar levels of homophobic and negative responses from healthcare providers in those settings.

Gay men and lesbians live in a society in which no protection in law is afforded to them as a direct result of discrimination related to their sexual orientation at work, in housing or health-care. Yet in this last situation, and particularly where their GP is concerned, one would hope to find a more sympathetic view. After all, this could have direct healthcare consequences. If, for example, a gay man was unknowingly infected with HIV, and began taking some of the early symptoms of the disease to a GP, it would be important for that GP to be aware of any possible HIV exposure. It is agreed that early identification, monitoring and management of HIV disease results in longer and improved quality of life, and GPs have been called on to play a key role in this. A holistic grasp of the individual's total lifestyle should be part of the healthcare provider's remit to deliver services appropriate to people's needs. In the case of gay men, we would suggest that the homophobia they experience in so many other areas of their life should not be evident in the healthcare setting. As the first port of call for most people is their primary healthcare practitioner, GPs in particular should be sympathetic to and conscious of the health needs of gay men (see McColl 1994, Schwartz 1994).

Conclusion

Health promotion for gay men has, understandably in recent years, focused exclusively on their risks of contracting and transmitting HIV and other sexually transmitted infections. However, particular aspects of gay men's lives put them at risk of other health problems to the same or greater extent than comparable heterosexual men. There is certainly scope for those wishing to see an improvement in gay men's health to target health promotion activities at alcohol and smoking, and for efforts to be directed at men using illicit drugs on the dance scene.

Gay men are still subject to violent attack and intimidation despite apparently more liberal attitudes, particularly among young people, to homosexuality. Paradoxically, reduced social stigma may result in more men coming out, and their greater visibility could result, in the short term at least, in more frequent physical attacks. Gay men appear to be at increased risk of mental health problems when compared with their heterosexual counterparts.

Reports of homophobia in healthcare settings suggest that it remains unwise in many situations for men to come out as gay, and so the full range of gay men's health needs will remain ill-understood until there is a change in this situation and appropriate studies have been carried out. Gay men do not seek special treatment with regard to the health problems that they face, merely equality of opportunity to maintain a healthy lifestyle and to have access to healthcare that is of a standard comparable to that offered to their heterosexual peers.

References

Bhugra D 1987 Homophobia: a review of the literature. Sexual and Marital Therapy 2(2):169–177

Bux D A 1996 The epidemiology of problem drinking in gay men and lesbians – a critical review. Clinical Psychology Review 16:277–298

Chaimowitz G A 1991 Homophobia among psychiatric residents, family practice residents and psychiatric faculty. Canadian Journal of Psychiatry 36:206–209

Coyle A 1993 A study of psychological well-being among gay men using the GHQ-30. British Journal of Clinical Psychology 32:218–220

Coyle A, Daniels M 1993 Psychological well-being and gay identity: some suggestions for promoting mental health among gay men. In: Trent D R, Reed C (eds) Promotion of mental health, vol 2. Avebury, Aldershot

Daling J R, Weiss N S, Klopfenstein L L, Cochran L E, Chow W H, Daifku R 1982 Correlates of homosexual behaviour and the incidence of anal cancer. Journal of the American Medical Association 247:1988–1990

Erwin K 1993 Interpreting the evidence: competing paradigms and the emergence of lesbian and gay suicide as a 'social fact'. International Journal of Health Services 23:437–453

Key issues for practitioners

- Gay and bisexual men have been ill served by general health research.

- Gay men are not only exposed to the same health risks as heterosexual men, but also to gay-specific risks e.g. mental health problems, higher rates of attempted suicide, higher levels of violence.

- The gay scene itself may contribute to ill health through high intake of alcohol, tobacco and illicit drugs.

- Gay men face problems of homophobia in healthcare services.

- Health promotion has focused understandably on risks of HIV and other STIs amongst gay and bisexual men but other health needs tend to be ignored.

Practical pointers

- Health promotion activities could usefully be targeted at alcohol and smoking and the use of illicit drugs on the dance scene.

Fitzpatrick R, Dawson J, Boulton M, McLean J, Hart G, Brookes M 1994 Perceptions of general practice among homosexual men. British Journal of General Practice 44:80–82

Flowers P, Smith J A, Sheeran P, Beail N 1998 'Coming out' and sexual debut: understanding the social context of HIV risk-related behaviour. Journal of Community and Applied and Social Psychology 8:409–421

French S A, Story M, Remafedi G, Resnick M D, Blum R W 1996 Sexual orientation and prevalence of body dissatisfaction and eating disordered behaviours – a population-based study of adolescents. International Journal of Eating Disorders 19:119–126

Gettleman T E, Thompson J K 1993 Actual differences and stereotypical perceptions in body-image and eating disturbance – a comparison of male and female heterosexual and homosexual samples. Sex Roles 29:545–562

Gibson P 1989 Gay male and lesbian youth suicide. In: Report of the Secretary's task force on youth suicide, vol 3: Prevention and interventions in youth suicide. DHHS Publications 89–1623, US Government Printing Office, Washington DC

Gold R 1995 Why we need to rethink AIDS education for gay men. AIDS care 7 (S1):S11–S19

Goodkin K, Blaney N T, Tuttle R S et al 1996 Bereavement and HIV infection. International Review of Psychiatry 8:201–216

Hart G, Fitzpatrick R, McLean J, Dawson J, Boulton M 1990 Gay men, social support and HIV disease: a study of social integration in the gay community. AIDS Care 2:163–170

Hart G J, Dawson J, Fitzpatrick R M, Boulton M, McLean J, Brookes M, Parry J V 1993 Risk behaviour, anti-HIV and anti-hepatitis B core prevalence in clinic and non-clinic samples of gay men in England, 1991–1992. AIDS 7:863–869

Hart G J, Flowers P, Der G J, Frankis J S 1999 Gay men's HIV-related sexual risk behaviour in Scotland. Sexually Transmitted Infections 75:242–246

Herek G M, Gillis J R, Cogan J C, Glunt E K 1997 Hate crime victimisation among lesbian gay, and bisexual adults – prevalence, psychological correlates, and methodological issues. Journal of Interpersonal Violence 12:195–215

Jay K, Young A 1979 The gay report: lesbians and gay men speak out about sexual experiences and lifestyles. Summit Books, New York, pp 729–731

Johnson A M, Gill O N 1989 Evidence for recent changes in sexual behaviour in homosexual men in England and Wales. Philosophical Transactions of the Royal Society of London Series B – biological sciences 325:153–161

Kitzinger C, Coyle A 1995 Lesbian and gay couples: speaking of difference. The Psychologist February:64–69

Mann M, Tarantola D J M, Netter T W 1992 AIDS in the World. Harvard University Press, Cambridge MA

McColl P 1994 Homosexuality and mental health services. British Medical Journal 308:550–551

Macintyre S 1992 The effects of family position and status on health. Social Science and Medicine 35:453–464

Mason A, Palmer A 1996 Queer Bashing. Stonewall, London

Meyer I H 1995 Minority stress and mental health in gay men. Journal of Health and Social Behaviour 36:38–56

Nord D 1996 The impact of multiple AIDS-related loss on families of origin and families of choice. American Journal of Family Therapy 24:129–144

Rotheram-Borus M J, Hunter J, Rosario M 1995 Coming out as Lesbian or gay in the era of AIDS. In: Herek G M, Greene B (eds) AIDS identity and community. Sage, London

Schatz B, O'Hanlon K 1994 Anti-gay discrimination in medicine: results of a national survey of lesbian, gay and bisexual physicians. American Association of Physicians for Human Rights, San Francisco

Schwartz G R 1994 Getting to know your patients and peers. Journal of the American Medical Association 271:712

Simms I, Hughes G, Swan A, Rogers P, Catchpole M 1998 New cases seen at genitourinary medicine clinics: England 1996. Communicable Disease Review 8:S1–S11

Skinner W F 1994 The prevalence and demographic predictors of illicit and licit drug use among lesbians and gay men. American Journal of Public Health 84:1307–1310

Unlinked Anonymous Surveys Steering Group 1998 Unlinked anonymous HIV prevalence monitoring programme, England and Wales, Data to end 1996. Department of Health, London

21

Testicular cancer: no laughing matter?

Lesley Hamilton

Introduction

A famous comedian once said he'd heard that there was a national campaign to get men to examine their testicles more frequently .... However, he couldn't understand why there needed to be a campaign – all the men he knew examined their testicles every 5 minutes and would know if they had a new hair growing, let alone a lump!

The audience laughed, but for many of them this was far from a laughing matter. Each year some 1500 men in England and Wales develop testicular cancer. In 1996, 68 men died from the disease, 46 of them aged between 15 and 44 (OPCS 1997). They die needlessly because testicular cancer is a disease that, if treated promptly, can be cured. Unfortunately many of these men, contrary to popular opinion, don't examine their testicles, or if they do, they ignore any changes that they find. They die from embarrassment or ignorance because no-one told them how important it is to get to know their own bodies, recognise when something is going wrong and to seek help as soon as possible.

So why do we laugh at the thought of men examining their testicles? Men's health is a joke in itself to some people. The view that men aren't interested in health promotion or disease prevention is prevalent among health professionals. Certainly it's often said that there's no point in trying to discuss such things with men, and perhaps the conventional approaches to these issues are not appropriate for them. When did you last see a group of men chatting about vitamin supplements or how often you should have your eyes tested? It's likely that any mention of eyesight will probably be more centred on the needs of a particular football referee than the needs of the men themselves. So are we, as health professionals, missing the point? Personal experience in both my private and professional life tells me that men are interested in health and they do want information, so why do we still laugh at the very idea of health promotion messages for men? Where are we going wrong?

Local background

In Northamptonshire in 1992 we were faced with trying to find some way of addressing these difficulties as part of a local

health promotion campaign to raise awareness of the importance of self-examination and early detection of cancer. It
became clear that there was a general lack of knowledge about
testicular cancer among professional groups locally. Many staff,
both male and female, expressed embarrassment at the thought
of raising such a sensitive issue and expressed reservations
about teaching an individual to examine their own testicles.

These issues had to be addressed if we were going to succeed
in our attempts to encourage men to come forward for help and
advice. We decided to provide training and resources to support
professionals in this new role before we began to raise public
awareness.

Epidemiology of testicular cancer

Testicular cancer was a very rare disease at the beginning of this
century, with fewer than 60 deaths recorded in the UK each
year. However, incidence has increased dramatically since then.
In 1982, 843 new cases were registered in England and Wales.
In 1992, the number was 1382 and lifetime risk of developing
the disease testicular cancer was 1 in 480. In the US, incidence
has doubled since the 1930s, and is continuing to increase
(Kincade 1999).

The aetiology of the disease is unknown, but two main factors
appear to be related to incidence:

1. *Age* – testicular cancer is a disease of young men. It is the
   most common solid tumour in men aged 15–34.
2. *Cryptorchidism* – where there is a history of one undescended testis the lifetime risk increases to 1 in 120. This
   rises to 1 in 44 where there is a history of two undescended
   testes.

Incidence of testicular cancer varies considerably. In England,
rates range from 4.5 per 100 000 population in North East
Thames to 7 in Oxford and 7.4 in Wessex. Rates in northern
European countries differ by a factor of nearly 10 (Adami et al
1994). Data from America show that it is more common in
higher socioeconomic groups (Kincade 1999) and 5 times more
common in white than black populations (Bosl & Motzer
1997). Epidemiological and biological evidence indicates that
the factors influencing the development of this cancer act early

in life, possibly before birth (Kristensen et al 1996). In some countries there is an association with dairy product consumption and testicular cancer (Davies et al 1996). Trauma and infection have also been suggested as causative factors, but no actual links have been established.

The local campaign

The lack of knowledge about the cause of the disease can have both a positive and a negative effect on health promotion messages. On the one hand men may perceive that there is nothing they can do to reduce their risk of testicular cancer, so why should they worry about it? On the other hand the message is very clear: all men are at risk of developing the disease, so all men should learn to examine themselves. What makes the testicular cancer message so important is that 90% of cases can be cured if detected and treated early (Stavda & Stentella 1983). The campaign we designed focused on this very powerful message. The slogan we chose reflected this: 'Testicular self-examination saves lives'.

Aims of the campaign

The main aim of the campaign was to raise public and professional awareness of the importance of testicular self-examination. We planned a comprehensive training programme for health professionals, produced an educational resource for use with the public, purchased a range of teaching aids and fact files for professionals and planned a major media event with the local rugby football team. We also supported each individual attending the training so they could develop this area of work in their own practice and provided free resources for public campaigns and displays.

The training

Training was offered as one of four modules in a programme designed to support the *Europe Against Cancer* initiative. We deliberately used an existing campaign as it was felt unlikely that health professionals would attend training on a single issue like testicular cancer. The other three modules were:

1. breast cancer
2. cervical cancer
3. making an action plan – supporting individuals to incorporate this new information into their work.

It seemed important to include female cancers since women make up the majority of the caseload for many community nurses, and they may not have chosen to attend a men's health-oriented training session. In fact many of the trainees identified this as an issue during the training and developed strategies to use their existing contact with women to pass the message on to men. Others realised that they could expand their opportunities to work directly with men.

Recruitment

We advertised the training 3 months in advance, sending flyers out to all primary healthcare team managers, GP practices, Acute and Community Trusts and occupational health nurses. Each module was offered twice, over a period of 2 weeks, alternating mornings and afternoons to allow the greatest flexibility of attendance. This approach and the long lead-in to the training were appreciated by managers, who were able to organise off-duty rotas well in advance.

Attendance

A total of 89 people attended the training including:

- school nurses
- health visitors
- practice nurses
- occupational health nurses.

Each participant completed an action plan, which we kept a copy of. We wrote to each course participant 1 month after the training asking how they were progressing with their action plan and offering support. Very few needed any help; where it was requested, it was mainly regarding resources.

Resources

We designed and produced a leaflet and poster aimed at raising the awareness of the general public, which described in detail how to carry out self-examination. We chose a sporting theme which linked with our main public event, and also reinforced the positive health message we were trying to get across. These resources were made available at no cost to anyone in the Health Authority area, and were offered for sale nationally. Since the campaign these resources have been updated and sales to other areas subsidise continued free local provision.

We purchased and made available through our free resource lending library a range of videos, models of testicles and other teaching aids. These included a flip chart with diagrams and information about testicular cancer and self-examination. Those health professionals who were lacking in confidence about raising this issue found this particular resource extremely useful since it provided them with a 'crib sheet' and also allowed both client and professional to avoid eye contact. Usually this would be seen as having a negative effect on communication, but in some circumstances it can enable the practitioner to gain confidence when working in an unfamiliar and sensitive topic area, and provide a less threatening approach for the client.

Media coverage

Once we had completed the training we felt it was important to give the campaign some impetus by using the local media. We approached the local rugby football team who were doing very well in the league. The team agreed to support us and a series of initiatives were planned. We first equipped the team doctor, a local GP, with the information and resources to run training sessions for all the team members, including the players, youth teams, coaches, physiotherapists and groundsmen. This was given coverage in the local evening and free papers under the headline 'Saints learn new ball skills'. This theme of innuendo and jokiness, although not generated by us, continued throughout the campaign, and seemed to allow men to overcome their initial embarrassment and talk about this sensitive issue. Further media coverage was given to the main public event.

Public campaign

Early in October 1992 we took our testicular self-examination (TSE) message to a high profile match attended by approximately 7000 supporters, the majority of whom were men. Health promotion specialists stood at each entrance to the ground, dressed appropriately in a Saints kit (which was extremely large and smelled of embrocation) and offered leaflets to people as they came in. We gave out 5000 leaflets that day and all were received with interest. Men could be seen reading the leaflet while they waited for the match to start and one or two actually left their seats to thank us for bringing the information to their attention. Many stood and talked to us at the entrances. Some talked of their own experience of friends or relatives who had developed testicular cancer, some talked of the loss and grief of losing a loved one. We were astonished at the response. A check around the ground confirmed that people had kept the leaflets – a search of the bins revealed only one or two discarded ones.

The Health Promotion Department had sponsored the match ball for the day and the Manager took pride of place in the Directors' box, where she made sure they all received a copy of the leaflet. Two members of the club's youth team walked the pitch before the game with a large banner proclaiming 'Testicular Self-Examination – it saves lives' and the programme included a full page about testicular cancer and self-examination. The commentator agreed to talk about the need for self-examination and where to go for advice during the interval and we manned a stand to provide on-the-spot advice. In short, there was no possibility of anyone at the match not being aware of the message.

The Saints won their match, and the commentator spontaneously commented, as the crowd prepared to leave: 'if you haven't touched a ball today, go home and touch two tonight'. The crowd roared with laughter, but this time the joke wasn't on them for a change. They had all learned something, and so had we: men *are* concerned about health issues, they *are* open to information about disease prevention and they *do* want to talk about their fears.

Professional and public information

In addition to the public event the health promotion department mailed information on testicular cancer along with a small supply of leaflets and posters to a wide range of health professionals and public settings requesting that it be displayed. This included every GP, community nurse manager, school, health centre, and occupational health department in the country. As many men do not come into contact with health professionals, we targeted other settings where men gather, including libraries, swimming baths, scout groups, boys clubs, local football clubs and retail outlets that stocked sports wear. In retrospect we could have included working men's clubs and pubs. We have also gone on to include testicular self-examination in men's health sessions in local prisons and young offenders' institutions, and to record a number of local radio programmes.

Training outcomes

This major event started the ball rolling, as it were, for the trainees. At the end of October all course participants were asked for information on their progress. A total of 57 course participants were by then incorporating information on testicular self-examination into their work in some way. School nurses had timetabled sessions with all sixth formers, health visitors were including the information in parentcraft sessions, practice nurses had included it in new patient and well person checks. The information was being offered to both men and women – an important consideration since we know that often lumps are detected by partners. The local police force issued the information to everyone on the force (maintaining the jokey theme by naming individuals responsible for doing 'spot checks'), and an occupational health nurse with links with the territorial army managed to run sessions for several hundred men at a local training camp. For most of the trainees, this had become an issue that they would incorporate into all their work in the future. There were, however, some trainees who did not respond to follow-up.

What did we learn?

As a department we learned a lot about this type of work.

Working with men

- Try to get at least one man involved in your planning group: an initiative around men's health needs input from men.

- Men do not use healthcare services in the same way as women, so don't expect to get messages to them through traditional routes such as GP surgeries or health centres. Go to the places where men meet: sports settings, pubs and clubs, workplaces.

- Use a language and style that are appropriate for the men you are targeting. Men may not be familiar with medical jargon and terminology, so be prepared to use colloquial terms and to find ways of enabling men to articulate their concerns in their own way.

- Don't make any assumptions. We trained the male GP who worked with us on our campaign before he began working with men's groups. Testicular self-examination was not an issue he had addressed before, other than to give out leaflets.

- Men may have difficulty acknowledging they have symptoms or asking for help. Find ways of encouraging them to talk to each other about health issues.

- Be prepared to listen. The men we worked with wanted to talk and talk. They had no preconceived ideas or barriers and I felt we only addressed the tip of the iceberg when we raised the issue of testicular cancer.

- Consider new and innovative ways of getting your message across: are there any internet cafés in your area? Would the local college consider setting up a web page on TSE?

Training issues

- If you are offering training for health professionals you must get managers, training officers and/or clinical tutors on your side. Include them in the planning and scheduling and in any media coverage if possible. Their commitment will greatly influence recruitment and attendance, and also give you practical ideas about how to incorporate your health message into the everyday work of your trainees.

- Health professionals like coming to training courses, especially if they are about new ideas and concepts. What is much harder to achieve, or to measure, is a change in their work practice as a result of the training. Try and build into your programme ways of monitoring change of practice or initiatives developed, and make it clear that these are the aims of the training.

- Offer appropriate accreditation for the people you want to attract to your training. Consider certificates of attendance, PGEA approval for doctors, or ENB approval for nurses.

- Multidisciplinary groups are, in general, easier to manage and more effective for training purposes. However, if you want groups to 'action plan', make sure you group people appropriately.

- Plan enough time for follow-up of trainees – a personal phone call or even a visit might make all the difference to outcome.

Resources

- If you are designing resources, look round to see what is already available – there is no point in re-inventing the wheel. Consider whether you want the resource to have a local focus or whether you might want to market it to other areas. Should you include local phone numbers or contact addresses?

- Get at least two people to proofread your resources, press releases, etc., particularly where the topic or terminology is at all ambiguous. We printed 10 000 leaflets with the slogan 'Examine your testicles one a month' instead of 'once a month', and had a barrage of phone calls asking 'Which one?'. Fortunately the mistake added to the local publicity, but it could have been disastrous.

- Pilot your resource with the target group and ask for their comments. Fix a deadline for comments from other professionals and stick to it.

- Try using information technology to your advantage: put TSE information on screen savers or prompts on college computers, or on websites used by local sports clubs, motor racing enthusiasts or other male-interest groups.

General issues

- Liaise with clinical providers if you are encouraging the public to seek help from them, and make sure they have the necessary information first. Health professionals will not be amused by a patient brandishing an article stating leaflets can be obtained from GPs, health visitors or practice nurses, if they haven't been forewarned and given this information. Consider whether your message has resource implications for local providers.

■ Use the media to get your message across to the public, but make sure it is *your* message. Choose a local celebrity or successful group who are used to working with the media, and will be of local interest, but make sure your message remains the main focus.

Conclusions

Action

Incidence of testicular cancer is increasing in this country. We do not have clear information about the causes, and so cannot offer any advice to men about how to prevent the disease. What is vital, therefore, is that we take every opportunity to ensure that men are aware of the signs and symptoms of the disease and seek help promptly. To enable this to happen, health professionals must be well informed and react promptly by initiating appropriate referrals and treatment. Only with a combination of these two approaches can we hope to reduce the number of deaths from this disease. Testicular self-examination can save lives, but only if it is practised and only if signs and symptoms are acted on swiftly.

A model for future work?

The approach described in this chapter has since been used by us as a model for working on a variety of issues. It encourages alliance working and establishes consistent accurate health messages across a wide range of practitioners. Health promotion specialists are a limited resource and do not have continuous access to their local population. On the other hand practitioners working with a caseload or defined client group do have direct contact with large numbers of the population, but are often not able to spend time identifying specific health issues and designing health promotion programmes, producing good quality educational tools and researching client information. Working together we can all make the best use of our own skills, resources and opportunities.

What next?

Healthcare workers are constantly juggling new information and initiatives with their existing workload. The initial impetus for health messages can soon be lost, and we are aware of the continued need to keep practitioners up-to-date and testicular self-examination on the agenda. We have redesigned our leaflet, and review our educational resources on a regular basis. There does remain one cause for concern, however: although treatment for testicular cancer is very effective, prevention would be even better. There is a strong need for further research into the causes of this disease. While the incidence of testicular cancer continues to increase and we are unable to identify why, the joke will remain on us.

Key issues for practitioners

- A dual approach involving men themselves and health professionals is vital when addressing an issue like testicular cancer.
- Don't expect health messages to get to men through traditional routes such as GP surgeries or health centres. Go to the places men go to, e.g. workplaces, pubs and clubs and sports settings.
- Men have difficulty acknowledging symptoms or asking for help.

Practical pointers

- Try to ensure at least one man is part of the planning process.
- Provide training and support to professionals before engaging with the public, and offer accreditation and ways of monitoring initiatives.
- Use language appropriate to the men you are targeting.
- Listen to men – you may well find they want to talk.

References

Adami H-O, Bergstom R, Mohner M et al 1994 Testicular cancer in nine northern European countries. International Journal of Cancer 59:33–38

Bosl G, Motzer R 1997 Testicular germ cell cancer. New England Journal of Medicine 337:242–253

Cancer Research Campaign 1991 Testicular cancer factsheet. Cancer Research Campaign, London

Davies T, Palmer C, Ruja E, Lipscombe J 1996 Adolescent milk, dairy product and fruit consumption and testicular cancer. British Journal of Cancer 74:657–660

Kincade S 1999 Testicular Cancer. American Family Physician, May

Kristensen P, Anderson A, Irgens L, Bye A, Vagstad N 1996 Testicular cancer and parental use of fertilizers in agriculture. Cancer Epidemiology, Biomarkers & Prevention 5 (January):3–9

OPCS 1997 Mortality statistics, cause, England and Wales. HMSO, London

Stavda K, Stentella J 1983 Cancer prevention and detection: testicular cancer. Cancer Nurse 6(6):468–486

References

22

A suicide prevention strategy for young men

Brian MacKenzie

Introduction

This chapter describes the development and implementation of a local suicide prevention strategy in Dorset in the mid-1990s which has been shown to be successful. A similar model has since been used in relation to other issues.

Dorset and suicide

The county of Dorset on the south coast of England has a population of approximately 670 000. Half live in the densely populated conurbation of Poole and Bournemouth, and half in more rural areas, centred on market towns and small villages. Much of the west of the county is very sparsely populated, with Weymouth the only significant urban area.

The male suicide rate in Dorset has been slightly above the national average since the 1970s, but not significantly so. Nevertheless, this has been of interest to the Health Authority as, for almost all other causes of death, the standardised mortality rates are lower than the national rate.

The greatest rise in suicides in recent years has been in the younger age groups. This is in line with the national – and the international – trend, at least among most industrialised nations. A number of factors are believed likely to contribute to increasing male suicide rates in Dorset, including:

- divorce becoming much more common
- job opportunities for men continuing to decline, particularly in the traditional male work environments of defence, farming, labouring and construction
- the ratio of job vacancies to job seekers, which has been as high as 1:6 – amongst the highest in the UK
- in rural communities, the stereotyping of roles between the sexes remains strong
- the great changes in farming communities since the 1950s, with a continuous decline in the number of people employed in agriculture and farming becoming an increasingly isolated occupation. (A Wessex-wide audit of suicides between 1988 and 1993 confirmed that Dorset has a higher than average number of suicides amongst farmers and other agricultural workers.)

Because of this picture, it was decided during 1994 to focus on young men over a long period, and to develop a health promotion campaign aimed at encouraging them to talk about their problems. Focus groups were used to develop a media-led campaign in the immediate pre-Christmas period. Posters, beer mats (which three breweries agreed to use) and radio advertising acknowledged that men often find the hardest option is to talk about problems, rather than attempting to sort them out for ourselves. Our message was: 'You've got to be tough to tell someone what's up. Talk about your problems – that way they'll get sorted.'

The impact of such a presentation is of course difficult to gauge, but we do know that there was good penetration of the material. The launch featured on regional television news, and there was good coverage in the other media.

As we reflected on that campaign and sought to build on it during 1995, two random factors determined our progress.

1. We saw the resource materials for World Mental Health Day, and didn't like them
2. We had available a person who was able to do some project work.

We therefore asked ourselves how we could best devise a comprehensive local strategy for suicide prevention. We decided to issue an open invitation to everyone in Dorset with a professional interest in the subject to come to a conference on World Mental Health Day.

Conference structure

The conference was to provide both local and national perspectives on the issues, and allow time for participants to begin developing an action plan for Dorset. The project worker made all the arrangements and ensured that the presenters had a common understanding of the day's goals. The conference was structured as described below.

National and local perspectives
The range of experts included a professor of social work studies, a consultant child and adolescent psychiatrist, a clinical psychologist and a consultant in public health medicine.

Themed interdisciplinary workshops
The workshop themes were:

- Men, violence and criminality
- Promoting self-esteem in young men
- Promoting the mental health of young men in rural areas
- Drug and alcohol abuse

- Developing new lifeskills in young men
- Masculinity and fatherhood.

Each workshop lasted 90 minutes, and one or two people gave short presentations which were followed by general discussion. Two relatively short – but very powerful – presentations were given by people who had first-hand experience of suicide or deliberate self-harm. There was also a short presentation on young men's issues, looking at 'modern' (perhaps postmodern?) masculinity.

Settings-based workshops

Workers from the various settings – education and youth services; social services; criminal justice; NHS; the voluntary sector – were asked to reflect on the day's presentations, and to translate their discussions into priorities for the work agenda of each organisation. Individuals were also asked to make personal commitments for action.

Attendance

We had to stop registrations when we got to 200, because the fire regulations for the venue wouldn't let us take any more. Those who came were from a very wide range of disciplines and interest groups, and covered as good a spread of Dorset's services as we could have wished.

From talk to action

Following the production of the conference report, we reflected on the suggestions for action made in the presentations and workshops, together with what we knew from the literature. From this material, an action plan was drafted which assigned lead agency responsibility to the actions. This plan was taken through the agencies by people who had been at the conference, and the final plan was owned by the agencies. Initially monitored by the Health Authority, this role was taken over by the Integrated Youth Purchasing Group which was established in the wake of the 1996 local government reorganisation, as a result of one of the conference recommendations.

The plan was laid out following the framework of the Ottawa Charter for Health Promotion, which says that effective health promotion requires that we:

- build healthy public policy
- create supportive environments for healthy behaviour
- strengthen community action
- develop personal skills
- reorient the health services.

The themes that emerged from the conference and people's ideas for moving things forward, fell into a number of distinct areas, as outlined below.

Mental illness

It is estimated that 25–30% of all suicides in the United Kingdom are committed by people with severe mental illness. A number of the ideas to emerge from the conference related to improving services for this group of people.

Drugs

Drug and/or alcohol misuse is a major risk factor for suicide. Action in this area has been linked to the *Tackling Drugs Together* initiative.

Isolation

Many other ideas tied in with the work of other major alliance groupings in Dorset, particularly the Rural Development Partnership for Dorset and Single Regeneration Bid initiatives.

For young people, isolation can be a real problem and until recently there have been very few social opportunities for them local to their own area. This is changing with the development of what are known as 'One-Stop Shops', otherwise called Young Persons' Advisory Services. These combine a social facility, in the form of a meeting place in a café-type atmosphere, with access to help and advice on a number of issues, such as:

- homelessness or housing difficulties
- relationship problems
- sexual health questions
- substance misuse concerns
- difficulties in accessing employment or training.

By January 2000 there were 12 One-Stop Shops in operation in Dorset, with two more being planned. These represent local alliances, particularly involving Health and Youth Services, but also local people. Although they have similar aims and objectives, the range of services offered by each One-Stop Shop is very much linked to local needs.

Prisons

There are four prisons in Dorset, taking sentenced prisoners from across the country. A therapeutic community was opened at Portland Young Offenders' Institute in April 1997 to improve the social skills and the resistance of young offenders to drugs. Drug-free wings have been established at the Verne and Dorchester prisons.

Work

As major local employers, the statutory services such as the NHS, Social Services, the police and the Probation Service, could do a great deal to alter male stereotypes. Two ways of doing this would be to:

1. actively seek to reduce the long working hours culture
2. provide better paternity leave arrangements.

Schools

The Dorset Education Partnership links health education in schools across a number of key areas such as drugs awareness, sexual health and increasingly, mental health. The development of coping skills, assertiveness and understanding life stages are seen as being key to good mental health. Programmes on managing bullying are offered to teachers, and preparation for parenthood modules are currently being trialed in secondary schools.

Where are we now?

The action plan which resulted from the conference included 28 objectives and 49 specific actions involving nine separate agencies. All but three actions – which relate to supporting the increased participation of fathers in all aspects of care for their children – have been achieved and/or are ongoing. Various partnerships in Dorset continue to press forward on a number of agendas which should impact on individual suicide risks. They include:

- the Drug Action Team
- Rural Development and Single Regeneration Bid Partnerships

- work with the criminal justice system
- the continued development of One-Stop Shops
- the work of the Dorset Education Partnership.

A guide for the media has been produced to encourage sensitive reporting of suicide, avoiding romanticising the act and encouraging the media to present the real facts, including not avoiding mention of mental illness where this is present. This guide was launched on World Mental Health Day 1996.

A county-wide Youth Strategy Group has been established to coordinate the development of services for young people across agencies, including the NHS, Social Services, education, Youth Services, the police and Probation Service, as well as the voluntary and independent sectors. This group monitors the implementation of the Suicide Prevention Strategy and also pools information on need across the county. Indicators of need include:

- numbers and locations of young people in contact with the criminal justice system
- those excluded from school
- concentrations of homelessness amongst young people
- areas with a high prevalence of substance misuse or teenage pregnancy.

The building-up of a profile from these indicators is allowing increasingly sensitive targeting of service development and prevent duplication of investment across agencies.

At the same time as the conference, we commissioned a theatre-in-education group to work with eight groups of Year 10 boys. The aim was to allow the boys to explore their attitudes to the idea of 'Depression', and to help them develop skills for coping in times of emotional distress. The report that came out of this work, called *What Boys Worry About*, makes for fascinating reading, and has been widely distributed throughout Dorset.

In 1997 work began in HealthWorks in conjunction with the three local Youth Services and three Samaritans branches with the aim of increasing the acceptability of the Samaritans to young people. The work included a media-led campaign of posters and credit-card-size information giving the local Samaritan phone numbers in a format (and using words) designed in close consultation with young people. The message was: 'Don't get down, get help. Any problem, any time. In confidence, round the clock.' A spin-off of this work is that the Youth Services and the Samaritans have had input into each others' training programmes, and two multi-agency training days on working with young people have been held.

GPs in Dorset have taken on board the *Defeat Depression* campaign. That has now extended into a more comprehensive training programme. Audit of deliberate self-harm services has resulted in:

- social workers being appointed to provide assessment at A & E departments
- the development of a standard assessment pro forma
- a rolling training programme in risk assessment for A & E staff, provided by specialist mental health services.

This completes our outline of what has happened in relation to suicide prevention and young men in Dorset since 1994. A full account of the actions taken can be found in the Action Plan document.

Has it worked?

When we began this work, the male suicide rate in Dorset was among the worst 10% in England and Wales. The latest figures available (to 1998) show that we have moved into the second 10%.

It is impossible to claim a causal relationship between the work that has been done and the change in our national position. Clearly, we have no way of knowing what would have happened if we had not acted. It is certainly the case that a lot has been achieved which is good in itself – such as fostering interagency collaboration and providing training for a range of professionals and volunteers – whether or not it ultimately impacts on suicide rates.

In our view, enough has been done to shift the burden of proof. We are confident that the process has worked for us, and that it is now reasonable to ask any sceptics to demonstrate that it was something else that has made the difference. We continue to assert that the process of holding a local conference leading to an implemented action plan is a powerful tool for translating talk into action. Its power derives from four key factors:

1. Local professionals are able to test their current beliefs and practice against what is known – nationally and internationally – about effective interventions.
2. An action plan is drawn up which allows each agency to be clear about what its contribution is to the whole agenda.
3. The actions get written into people's work programmes.
4. Progress is monitored and reported back to each agency.

We have replicated the process twice since 1995. The first time was during Child Safety Week in 1996, when we held a conference on the issues of data collection and effective interventions in relation to child accidents, and drafted an action plan. Unfortunately, the local government reorganisation process then got in the way, and the reality of getting agreement across three authorities with differing priorities and structures meant that implementation was shelved.

More successful was a February 1997 conference entitled 'What works in drugs education'. The action plan from that conference was picked up by the Drugs Action Team and its reference groups, and forms part of its ongoing programme.

With regard to our suicide prevention work, our challenge now is to revisit the implemented action plan, and make sure that the momentum is not lost. The young men of Dorset deserve no less.

Key issues for practitioners

- A multiagency approach using a conference as a starting point allowed professionals to test beliefs about what were effective interventions.

- Using action plans ensured each agency knew what its contribution to the work on suicide prevention would be.

Practical pointers

- One-Stop Shops offering informal meeting places with access to advice and help are closely linked to local young men's needs.

- A guide for the media helped to avoid romanticisation and represent the real facts when reporting suicides.

- A county-wide youth strategy helped to build a profile of young men's needs, and allow for sensitive targeting of services.

Part 3
Guidelines for practice

Part 2 of this book revealed a rich and varied range of experience and ideas about working with men around health issues. In Part 3 we attempt to highlight the major themes affecting practice that emerge from these contributions and from our review of issues affecting men and health in Part 1. We then look at how practice can be developed in different settings, with different groups of men and through different ways of working. Building on these themes we offer some guidelines which are intended to support the development of a more positive and structured approach to health promotion work with men.

Part 3
Guidelines for practice

23
Guidelines for practice
Neil Davidson

This chapter covers:

- Why? The rationale for men's health work
- What? The content of men's health work
- How? Ways of working on men's health

Introduction

From the rich variety of material in Parts 1 and 2 of this book, some important general themes can be identified. We will examine these in this chapter, beginning with the why, what and how of health promotion work with men.

Why? The rationale for men's health work

What emerges very clearly from Part 1 is that we *do* have a rationale for specific health work with men. Certainly there is plenty of debate about what men's health actually means, what is and is not included, and whether we are primarily working with the effects of nature or nurture. Now more than ever before we need clarity to ensure we avoid a succession of one-dimensional approaches. Despite the lack of consensus on definitions, since the Chief Medical Officer's 1992 detailing of the epidemiological data and call to action, a clear case for a focus on specific work with men has grown and gained legitimacy.

The Labour Government's public health approach has given a new impetus to practitioners and strategists and will require a framing of men's health which will have to go beyond the biological and take note of the social and psychological. This may provide a positive framework for the development of men's health or it may turn out to make the job more complicated (see

Kendal Ch. 4). What is significant for those interested in developing practice is that there are data to justify a focus and a potential wider framework into which men's health work can be placed. The practitioners who have contributed to this book as well as growing numbers of others we have talked to don't doubt the *need* for work on men's health, even if there is still plenty of scope for discussion on how, where, what and when.

There is work still to be done on refining our rationale, on clarifying our aims and objectives, and on fitting the work into the new public health context. However, justification of need should be less controversial now than ever before and this should help clear the way for a clearer and more systematic approach to developing practice.

What? The content of men's health work

We have good epidemiological data about men and their health. We have both morbidity and mortality data, as well as wider statistical information about how employment, crime and education impact on men's lives. And as was pointed out in Part 1, although we don't yet have research which can provide definite cause and effect answers, there is a growing body of evidence about men's health beliefs and behaviours. Certainly there is still debate about the definition of men's health centred around biology, individual beliefs and behaviours, and masculinity. And of course we now have a new public health context for work with men in he shape of the Government's *Our healthier nation* adding its own 'spin' to this debate.

All this might lead us to expect inactivity amongst practitioners because of confusion about what they are supposed to be working on. However, the examples illustrated in Part 2 suggest that some practitioners at least have had enough clarity about the boundaries of 'men's health' to get started. For most contributors what identifies men's health work is an understanding of men's conditioning coupled with an acknowledgement that they are not a heterogeneous group. In practice this often means taking time to find out what different men think and feel about their health (see Hoare and Walsh Ch. 6, Hart and Mays Ch. 11, Twardzicki and Roche Ch. 16, Bhavsar Ch. 18). This 'back to basics' attitude has helped build a pragmatic approach to the content of men's health work.

The range of practice examples described in Part 2 reinforce the view of Fletcher quoted in Chapter 1 that:

Men's health will be defined by whatever health workers say it is. If nurses demonstrating testicular self examination say they are doing 'Men's Health' then that is what will be associated with the name. If social workers running programs for perpetrators of domestic violence say they are involved in 'Men's Health' then this activity will come under the banner too.

What practice there is has often developed *in spite of* a lack of consensus or clarity about content. The consequence is that at the broadest level progress has been slow and sporadic and strategically we have failed to make much headway. Yet what both Parts 1 and 2 suggest is that we are currently in a better position than ever to marry the learning of individual practitioners illustrated here with a new strategic and policy context.

How? Ways of working on men's health

We concluded in Part 1 that men's beliefs and behaviours require us to have some understanding of masculinity and its impact on men's health. From this we made some suggestions for developing practice interventions (listed on pp. 26–28), which are reflected in the contributions made by practitioners in Part 2. Three general themes on how we can work best with men emerge from this:

1. having a positive approach
2. experimenting with methods
3. building strategies.

A positive approach

Running through all the contributions in this book is an emphasis on the need to take a positive approach to working with men. Traditionally men have been seen by professionals as either disinterested or problematic. Whilst it is true that men certainly put up barriers which damage their health and inhibit their use of services it is also the case that health services and practitioners need to adopt a more 'men-friendly' attitude. A positive approach allows professionals to engage with men, assess their needs and offer appropriate services.

This might mean for example taking the work to where men are as Robinson (Ch. 13) highlights when talking about the use of sport as a medium for reaching boys on health issues Hoare and Walsh (Ch. 6) show how health professionals often fail to engage positively with men simply because they lack confidence. In this case the introduction of a simple tool (pro-forma questionnaires) allowed workers to actively engage with men instead of accepting the traditional 'disinterested and uncooperative' label. Bhavsar (Ch. 18) too shows how a positive attitude allows health professionals to engage in a process of finding out what particular groups of men really want from health services.

Experimenting with methods

The contributors highlight the variety of possible ways of working with men. Traditionally we have expected men simply to fit into existing ways of working which have often taken little or no notice of their particular needs. Methods which may have worked for women and children have not been particularly appropriate when working with men. All the practitioners writing here have effectively started from scratch and developed or adapted their normal way of working.

One longstanding complaint of health workers is that some men don't use services as well as women. Hamilton (Ch. 21) argues that targeted publicity is critical if we are to engage with men on health issues. She describes how surprised she and her colleagues were at the high level of interest in testicular cancer when a rugby club was targeted. Getting health messages to men is obviously vital and Hamilton's work shows how an imaginative approach can pay off.

Brown (Ch. 7) and Massaro (Ch. 19) show that we may need to reassess and or reinvent the 'tools of the trade' in health work with young men. Resources for health education work are often geared to young women and may not transfer easily to use with young men. Young men's apparent disinterest in talking about their health may in part reflect the fact that the games, videos and other resources we have been using don't address their needs.

Building strategies

The lack of strategic approaches to men's health both at local and national level is a theme running through most of the contributions to this book. The new public health context requires a muti-faceted approach to men's health. The experimenting that has gone on at a local level with methods, new approaches and multi-disciplinary working has had an impact but as Kendall (Ch. 4) points out, without a broader policy this learning may be lost and the potential for real change in men's health greatly diminished.

Many of the contributors emphasise the need for a national approach and some see the current climate as being fertile for this. Kendall argues that the Government's new approach to health, pushing for local health strategies, provides a good context in which men's health initiatives could thrive. Others, such as Fletcher (Ch. 5) talking about the Australian experience, emphasise that practice has at times developed in spite of policy makers and in the face of fluctuating political commitment.

Fletcher also sounds a warning against thinking that men's health work could develop in a similar pattern to women's health, reminding us that there are significant differences and using the example that it's unlikely that there will be a comparable groundswell of demand from men themselves for a national policy.

Evaluation

In addition we should consider the question of evaluation. Griffiths (Ch. 2) reminds us that there are differences between men, and that men's health is a complex issue for strategists as well as practitioners. Hoare and Walsh (Ch. 6), Wilkins (Ch. 2) and Massaro (Ch. 19) are all well aware of the need to evaluate work in order to provide ammunition for developing policies. Again, because development hasn't and probably won't be 'consumer'-led, professionals need to make a strong case for the effectiveness of what they are doing. Conversely, as Hoare and Walsh and Neil (Ch. 3) suggest, more research is needed to feed into new practice initiatives, and this needs to be sanctioned by policy makers looking at the 'bigger picture'.

General guidelines

Having summarised some of the main issues raised by contributors we will now try to develop these to provide some general starting points for those considering a practical and strategic approach to work on men's health issues.

Clarity of purpose

Many of us working with men sense the possibility of change, but fail to set clear and realistic targets for what we can do. A pressure exists to 'sort men out' and it's all too easy to succumb to the urgency associated with this. Whilst we should certainly have high expectations of what men are capable of, we also need to be realistic about the part we can play.

The most likely pitfall in men's health work is the effect that unrealistic or incoherent aims will have on morale and persistence. Many workers start with a deeply felt pessimism about men's ability to change – 'boys will be boys' – which is also unrealistic. By setting clear and achievable aims and explicit outcomes we are far more likely to actually proceed with work and, significantly, to *maintain* it.

Although varied, the examples of practice in this book stand out because of their clarity of purpose. The temptation exists to try and 'change men' on a wider social level, but a clearly defined focus is essential. Twardzicki and Roche's work (Ch. 16), for example, picks out a particular health and safety issue – skin cancer; a particular group of men – outdoor workers; and a particular approach – participatory workshops on site. The aims are clear, the methods simple and targeted and thus the effectiveness of the work can be more easily evaluated.

The aims and outcomes of working with men on health issues need to be based on:

- our understanding of men and their health needs
- the barriers thrown up by men's conditioning and society's expectation of men's roles and behaviour
- our own skills, resources, motivation and an understanding of professional barriers
- the context in which we are working.

A few simple aims and outcomes regularly reviewed in the light of experience and changing understanding are far more likely to succeed than either an overoptimistic manifesto, or a pessimistic outlook which condemns workers to containing and limiting the damage done by men's behaviour and attitudes.

Understanding men

A basic factor inhibiting the development of work with men has been our lack of detailed knowledge of men's attitudes, behaviour and feelings about health. Comparatively little research has been done. We know little, for example, about how men make decisions on health matters or what influences them to visit the doctor for help. As a consequence those working in this field have to rely on what men themselves provide in the way of information.

As we have seen, many men's conditioning makes talking about health and contact with services difficult. What men present to the world, what they say and do in the *public* arena such as a health clinic is often very different to what may be happening in *private*.

A major consequence of men's reticence and silence is that the gap gets filled by assumptions, prejudices and stereotypes. Men don't talk – so we tend to generalise on the basis of the public front they present. As workers we need to break through this front and access the more private face of men's relationship with their health. This is central to developing work with men on these issues.

Not only do we need to find out more about men, it is also important that we check out our assumptions about them. The stereotypes we carry may create significant barriers to men's use of services. Acknowledging these is as important for men working in this field as it is for women.

The value of attempting to increase our knowledge of men cannot be underestimated. Hoare and Walsh's contribution (Ch. 6) highlights the value of deepening our understanding in order to build more effective practice interventions. Through preliminary research a new paradigm of understanding men's approaches to contraceptive use was discovered. The understanding of different approaches amongst men – opportunistic, passive, and prepared – allowed work to be much more specific and targeted according to need. This preparatory research also showed that our own assumptions as workers can be real barriers to men. We have made the point throughout this book that men are not a homogeneous group and that different approaches are needed. Hoare and Walsh's work illustrates this well.

In order to understand men and health we have to get to know, and perhaps improve our communication with, men. This should be the foundation for both increasing our knowledge of them and diminishing our reliance on stereotypes and assumptions. Box 23.1 lists some guidelines to help us to understand men better.

Box 23.1   Understanding men – some guidelines

- Read about men and what they say about health.

- Make a decision to engage with men on health issues and let them know you are interested both at a one-to-one level and as a service.

- Take the initiative in talking about health, but be sensitive to their conditioning as men.

- Listen carefully to what men are saying. Disinterest or hostility may be a mask or front behind which lie real concerns. Learn to 'read between the lines'.

- Learn to distinguish between how men present themselves in public and in private. Public behaviour around health may be guided by the need not to lose face, or fear of humiliation or exposure, or uncertainty over social and gender roles. Private behaviour is distinguished by a higher degree of safety, of feeling understood, of a sense of confidentiality, privacy and trust. With an understanding of how this works for particular men, a worker may be able to turn seemingly public experiences into more private ones, where men's defences, barriers and pretence may be lowered.

- Start afresh with each man or group of men, where possible dropping assumptions. Find out how this man's interest in his own health shows itself.

- Identify barriers, both internal (due to men's conditioning) and external (those existing within health services and wider social systems). Use this knowledge as a basis on which to plan a more positive approach to developing work on men's health.

Building a positive approach

Increased understanding of men's relationship with their health – including the physical, psychological and social aspects – will help us plan the form the work needs to take. But we also need to build from a *positive* foundation. With all other population groups we start from the assumption that we can help, that we have an obligation to provide appropriate services and that if we aren't we can do something about it. Unfortunately this assumption of positivity has not always existed in relation to men.

Here are some suggestions which may help to foster a new approach to working with men.

Assume men are interested

Casting off personal prejudices about men's lack of interest in health is a vital starting point for the work. If we feel negative or cynical about its potential then we will be sending this message out to men, thereby reinforcing the view that looking after their health is 'not for them'. We should start by assuming men may well be interested – despite surface appearances. Discovering the right context for this interest to be expressed in is critical. Robinson (Ch. 13) describes how an interest in football fitness provided a channel through which wider health issues could be explored. Hamilton's work on testicular cancer (Ch. 21) is another good example of holding a working assumption of interest despite a real lack of 'consumer demand'. The imaginative publicity campaign successfully found a setting in which men felt safe enough to simply pick up a leaflet on an important health issue.

Preparation

An important starting point for workers is the need to thoroughly examine our own ideas, assumptions and feelings about men and health. This helps clarify thinking, connect to motivation, and acknowledge and develop the ability to step back from any assumptions we may have about men in order to see what needs to be done. Although preparation is useful in kickstarting our practice, we can only really develop ideas, skills and enhance our motivation by *doing the work*, reviewing as we go.

As well as personal preparation, it may also be useful to take some time to discuss issues around working with men with colleagues and those to whom we are accountable. Any new area of work may be greeted with suspicion or a lack of understanding. Enthusiasm to start work like this is vital but it should be tempered by trying to ensure that interested groups (other workers, local communities, managers) know what is going on and are given the opportunity to support rather than attack it.

Listening to men

One of the major reasons for the lack of development of work around health is that it appears as if men aren't interested or willing to take responsibility for this aspect of their lives. Undoubtedly there is some truth in this view, the reasons lying in the nature of men's *conditioning*, in the beliefs and behaviours men have about their health. Yet it is also true that as workers in this field we have been unable to hear men's concerns or to understand behaviour which appears to be disinterested or even hostile, but which may well be a disguise or front covering up genuine concerns. A key skill, therefore, is to listen carefully to what men are saying and reading their behaviour carefully. Hoare and Walsh's work (Ch. 6) highlights the value of expending effort on researching men's health beliefs and behaviours.

On a wider level we need to assess men's health needs. Both commissioners and practitioners have failed to systematically use research and needs analysis to build practice in the way they have for other population groups, as Neil points out in Chapter 3. This isn't always easy and mistakes get made as Bhavsar describes (Ch. 18), but if we wish to progress then our knowledge base about men needs to grow.

Building new kinds of relationships with men

Men's comparative lack of contact with those working on health issues is clearly a major barrier to workers wanting to improve men's health. Men are often strangers to healthcare services, except when a crisis develops. Traditionally women have acted as gatekeepers for a family's health, and health workers have tended to try and reach men through women. What this means is that in a health context, a traditional approach of encouraging men to act as active 'consumers' of services probably won't work. We may need to start not only outside the traditional environments where health is normally discussed and services delivered, but also outside of the traditional expert–patient/client relationship.

Broader relationships with men may need to be worked on to build men's trust in workers enough so that more sensitive health issues can be discussed. Hart and Mays (Ch. 11) describes how a broader community approach may provide a route into men's health. Williams' account of a testicular cancer self-help group (Ch. 10) is another example of breaking down the traditional medical model approach and encouraging men themselves to take more responsibility for their health.

Men have traditionally been suspicious and unsure of those working in health-related services, and trust may have to be built up with particular groups of men, especially those with little or no history of contact with traditional health settings. Hart and Flowers (Ch. 20) show that even when a group of men (in this case gay and bisexual men) have contact with services, it may be limited by a range of assumptions and prejudices. So gay men are targeted around sexual health but wider health issues are ignored.

Giving information

One of the most inhibiting factors in men's conditioning around health is that we feel we have to give an impression of knowing everything we need to know. This makes learning hard for boys and men and presents a problem for those working on health issues. The difficulties, in terms of admitting ignorance and potentially losing face, for boys and men, means that workers may have to take the initiative in information giving rather than waiting to be asked. Unlike women, men will not tend to act as active consumers of health information except perhaps where this can be done anonymously. For example, men are known to be active users of telephone helplines for advice on matters such as sexual health. The telephone, of course, allows men to remain anonymous and in control of the situation.

Workers need to give information even if boys and men protest that they 'know it all already'. Obviously this must not be done in a heavy-handed or patronising way, or it will be counterproductive. An effective strategy is to let men know that information-giving is a matter of routine rather than any personal reflection on their ignorance or lack of experience. Hoare and Walsh (Ch. 6) describe one way of doing this. They built in a sexual history questionnaire into their initial contacts with male clients in STD clinics. This normalisation of both information giving and questioning allows men to use the safety of a formal and standard procedure to engage with sexual health issues.

On a wider level, information needs to be made available to men in the form of leaflets, posters and other media. What has not happened historically, is the *targeting* of health information to men. It has been assumed that they will pick up leaflets aimed at a general audience. This is often not the case and research suggests that health information needs to be written and designed in a particular way to be made more attractive and relevant to boys and men. Health practitioners with experience working with men and an understanding of their conditioning could usefully be involved in helping those who produce information in order to make it more likely that it reaches and is used by men. Brown (Ch. 7) describes how important this process is in the production of resources.

Taking the initiative

Because of men's private lack and public show of confidence around health, those interested in developing this work are going to have to take initiatives to push it forward. This doesn't however mean dragging men somewhere they don't want to go. Rather, it means that as workers we have to be willing to raise issues first, to ask questions, and to persist with men until we get behind any front that exists.

Taking opportunities when men are receptive

There are key times when men's reluctance to look at their health diminishes or drops away entirely, including:

- at times of high levels of responsibility
- at times of crisis.

At times of high levels of responsibility, such as impending or recent fatherhood, men are often highly motivated towards thinking about their own and their family's wellbeing. Practically it is also a time when men are much more likely to be in contact with health-based organisations and have a legitimate reason for visiting them. Clinic workers or health visitors use this opportunity to encourage women to consider their own health and wellbeing, as well as their child's. There is no reason why this should not be extended to fathers as well.

At times of crisis, such as ill health, bereavement, relationship breakdown or unemployment, men are often more vulnerable and open, and more likely to seek help. A man with even a temporary disability from illness or injury may find himself questioning his role, attitudes, feelings and behaviour about all sorts of issues including his 'manhood'. Williams' description of setting up the self-help group Mind Over Matter (Ch. 10) is a good example of the potential for reaching men when a health crisis strikes. The difficulties they have had in sustaining contact with men beyond the initial crisis illustrates how much there is still to be done by health services in terms of a systematic approach to men's health.

The changing social and economic climate means that men's roles and identity are being questioned and accompanied by increased levels of stress and mental health problems. These problems tend to mean men are more likely to come into contact with those working on health issues and so could be significant turning points in their attitudes towards their health if our responses as workers are positive.

Training and support

Workers need more than just ideas and information. We may also need the opportunity to talk through our practice, our aims and our understanding. Training and support are key elements. Hoare and Walsh (Ch. 6) and Hamilton (Ch. 21) all built the training of professionals into a multifaceted approach to work on contraception and testicular cancer respectively, seeing the long-term benefits of bringing colleagues on board. Training can give us the opportunity to clarify our thinking and check out our assumptions and feelings, and is vital if we are to address our own professional barriers. Having time to reflect on new and sometimes difficult issues can be very valuable.

Experimenting

On a personal level a real barrier to the development of health work with men may lie in our own hesitance to get started.

Needing more understanding or more training or better resources may all seem like good reasons for not initiating projects, but in reality none of these need be a real barrier. We need to be prepared enough to get going, but the rest we can learn as we go. There is no blueprint for successful work with men – only a willingness to try things out and to keep thinking about what we are doing.

Multidisciplinary working

Thinking about what needs to happen for men at a wider strategic level means that new initiatives are much more likely to survive, prosper and be effective. This means considering the bigger picture of men's health, and at a local level this involves forging alliances with other agencies and organisations whose work impacts on men's health. Providing health clinics for men, for example, is important but these are likely to be far better used if boys and young men receive appropriate health education which encourages them to use such facilities. MacKenzie (Ch. 22) describes how concern about young men's suicide rates was translated into a multiagency suicide prevention strategy which fed into the action plans of a range of agencies. This approach prevents possible duplication of services and allows for increased sensitivity of targeting. Other contributors, including Robinson, Hamilton and Wilkins (Chs 13, 21 and 12), emphasise the importance of approaching men's health as a multidisciplinary issue.

Evaluation

Several contributors note that we also need to be evaluating the work we do so that we can provide those who commission or plan policy with the information they require to justify funding. Yet to date we have very little in the way of examples of evaluated practice in the field of men's health. Clearly this is a problem and one which will need a solution soon if men's health work is to progress in a climate in which effectiveness needs to be proved.

Guidelines

The examples of practice we have included in Part 2 show how varied the starting point and approach to work with men can be. We will now consider more specific applications of our general themes, looking at how practice can best be developed within approaches which focus on:

- different functions of health work,
- different settings
- different groups of men
- different conditions.

We will examine the barriers that are likely to exist for men themselves and for workers, and the opportunities and starting points for developing the work.

Two barriers which seem to cut across all the specific areas we will explore below are worth mentioning straight away:

1. The lack of both local and national strategic frameworks for men's health is clearly an inhibiting factor for many workers. Where they lack confidence or strong motivation, this policy gap can hold back the development of work.
2. Training and resources support (for example in the form of appropriate materials) are still lacking, and in a new area of work like this may well be critical in determining whether, for instance, a practice nurse or community workers feels able to start targeting men on health issues.

Health work functions

Primary care

Although primary care is the most public face of health, the facts highlighted in Part 1 show that men are generally poorer users of these services than women. We explored earlier why this might, suggesting that men's conditioning inhibits many of them from asking for help, or leads them to ignore or delay dealing with symptoms of illness. Barriers exist within many men which make visiting the doctor an unattractive prospect. Certain groups of men, such as younger and single men, are among the most infrequent users.

Yet it was also suggested in Part 1, as well as by Fletcher (Ch. 5), Jewell (Ch. 14) and Hart and Flowers (Ch. 20) in Part 2, that primary care services themselves put up barriers, albeit usually unintentionally, to men. Services have been designed primarily with the needs of women and children in mind. This historically determined structure is compounded by professionals' lack of knowledge of men's health needs or their lack of confidence about working with them.

However, there are a number of possible ways in which we might begin to improve men's relationship with primary care services. These are described in Box 23.2.

Box 23.2   Ways to improve men's relationship with primary care services

- Staff training and support will build knowledge and confidence about men's needs and the positive approaches which will encourage more frequent and appropriate use of services.

- Most health workers try hard to ensure that confidentiality and privacy are maintained for all the people they work with. For men, this may be critical in terms of their willingness to seek help in the first place. Privacy needs to be maximised where at all possible. For example, men often feel embarrassed sitting in public waiting areas where they can be seen to 'have a problem'. Appointment systems minimise waiting. Let men know exactly how your confidentiality rules operate – don't wait for them to ask.

- Place leaflet information racks and posters in private areas such as toilets as well as public ones so that men can pick up leaflets or read information without being seen by others.

- Many primary care environments have information and posters on health issues which not only give specific information but also let users know that the service is for them. Most of these materials tend to be aimed at women and/or children. A lack of appropriate images in posters or leaflets adds to men's expectation that health-related services are not for them. Where at all possible, seek out information which men can relate to.

- Many men complain that services run at times when they cannot attend. Consider the possibility of changing times to suit men's working hours.

- Open services for all may also be an inhibiting factor for some men. Men-only clinics or opening times may be a useful way of targeting men and of sending the message that the service is for them too (see Watson, Ch. 15).

Box 2.2   Cont'd

■ In order to overcome men's perception that services are not for them it may be necessary to look at how services are advertised. Do they explicitly include men, spelling out that they are welcome? If not, men will tend rightly or wrongly, to assume the opposite. If men are targeted by advertising, what messages are being given out? From what is known about men's conditioning it seems that practical, concrete services are paramount in encouraging men's involvement. A practically based service – condom distribution for example – may attract men more than advertising an all purpose 'Men's Clinic'. Men often, initially at least, respond better to specific service provision but will then let themselves use more general help once they are sure it is 'safe'. Men are likely to present with a practical problem and then move on to more emotional issues, so practical services provide a starting point for more social and emotional issues to be discussed.

■ Consider means of getting feedback from men about what they are being offered and what they want from healthcare.

■ If men still don't come, then target through specific services. Watson's description of setting up a Well Man Clinic in London is a good example of this, and of the variety of strategies that may be needed to attract men to healthcare services and keep them coming.

Health promotion and health education

Health promotion and education have faced many of the same barriers as primary care in relation to men's access. Women have long been willing consumers of health education messages and workers have become accustomed to running groups or campaigns or producing materials on women's and children's health. Unsurprisingly, men have appeared to be resistant to health promotion messages and unwilling students of health education. Again, to a certain extent those working in this field have had to contend with some men's difficulty in seeking help, in admitting to fears or ignorance or simply with their absence from settings where health education takes place. Stereotypes, fears and a lack of knowledge of men may persist, often leading to workers being unable to adapt their methods, materials and strategies to men's needs.

Despite this, health promotion and education have been fertile ground for some of the most significant initiatives in the development of work on men's health. Men have been targeted for initiatives about coronary heart disease and men's cancers.

One of health promotion's important functions is to find out about the health needs of the client groups they work with. Until recently men have not been seen as a separate client group. The work described by Hoare and Walsh in Chapter 6, and underlined by Kendall (Ch. 4), shows how important this needs analysis function is in shaping a service or a campaign. Their work revealed new information about men's attitudes to contraception, which formed the foundation for work supporting professionals and targeting health messages at men.

Access to men has been an issue historically for health workers, but health promoters and educators are in a good position to take the message to men rather than waiting for men to come to the message. Hamilton (Ch. 21) shows how this can be done in a particularly creative way. Taking a health message about testicular cancer to a setting where men already are (a rugby match) proved to be a successful and surprisingly straightforward approach. This context gets men on their home ground with their friends and the message can be put over in a light-hearted but effective way.

Fletcher too (Ch. 5) describes several Australian initiatives where the message travels to where men already are. The difficulties of access and men's resistance are diminished by this approach.

Reframing a health message is also important if we are to get information to men. It is not always the case that health educators have got the wrong information for men. It may be simply that the way it has been presented fails to take into account men's health beliefs and behaviours. Wilkins (Ch. 12) and Robinson (Ch. 13) both show how well-known connections between diet and health can be reframed so that men can apply them to their own concerns. In the first case this was through encouraging a team approach to weight loss, using men's desire to avoid standing apart from their peers. Robinson reframes the message by highlighting the fitness benefits of diet change within the context of a much loved activity – football.

Counselling and mental health

Men have been particularly reluctant users of services which address emotional and mental health issues. Many men's traditional stiff upper lip, or emotional illiteracy as it is now being termed, makes it even harder for them to seek help for a mental health problem than a physical one. Rising suicide rates amongst young men and high rates of alcohol and drug dependency suggest that many men delay seeking help when they have emotional difficulties, or divert the problem into the physical arena. As a consequence workers such as counsellors, who deal with psychological ill health, have tended to see far fewer men – except perhaps when they are brought along by women partners. The climate is changing, as Keshet-Orr reports (Ch. 8), but work with men in this area remains much less developed than in crisis services.

Even where the problems of male mental health have been recognised, many workers have felt unable to access men. Many of the assumptions and lack of confidence highlighted above also exist around men and emotions. As Keshet-Orr points out, many in this field have not asked men what it is they want from the service, what ways of working suit them. The tendency, once again, has been to fit men into pre-existing patterns which seemed to work well for women.

Opportunities do exist and several of our contributors have shown how the apparent barriers between men and mental health professionals can be overcome. Men's apparent reluctance to talk about their emotions is less apparent if a safe entry point is found. Sex, for example. Most men want a good sex life and if problems occur they are often highly motivated to sort them out. Keshet-Orr's contribution shows how willing men are to tackle their difficulties once contact has been made. Not only does concern about sex bring men into counselling, but it often allows them to explore other emotional issues once the overtly physical or dysfunctional problem has been addressed. Another entry point is described by Hart and Mays (Ch. 11), who show how once a group of men were comfortable talking about physical health issues, they were able to move on to more emotional ones. What both these examples reinforce is that many men *are* both concerned about their emotional lives and able to address mental health issues if their presenting concerns and interests are first acknowledged.

Thinking about the influences underlying men's health beliefs and behaviours also forces us to think about new ways of reaching them on emotional issues. Although there is much work yet to be done in this area, the use of telephone helplines can bridge the gap between needing support for emotional issues and having difficulty accessing it publicly. Fletcher (Ch. 5) gives a good example of this from Australia. We know that men tend to be good users of general helplines, which give them control over their help-seeking and anonymity. It may be that helplines or other anonymous routes such as e-mail and websites could open up services and health education to men.

Resources and the media

Until recently men generally were simply not targeted with health messages, either through specific health promotion and education materials or through the commercial media. The importance of producing material which addresses the needs of particular groups has long been recognised by health professions and others, and gradually those groups marginalised from generic health work have been targeted. However, health workers have tended not to consider men as a marginalised group. The complaint has long been that men won't read leaflets or act preventatively to protect their health. Whilst this has probably been true there is a growing recognition that, in private at least, many men are interested in finding out more about their health. The difficulty for workers has not only been the reluctance to target materials in terms of form and content, but also the perceived difficulty of access, of actually getting the materials to men.

Brown (Ch. 7) reiterates these problems and suggests a number of ways workers might begin to match health information to men, and in particular to acknowledge the different needs of different groups of men. Knowing the intended audience's needs, and the formats and styles of resource they find attractive is critical. If men don't see themselves as an audience for health materials then we need to start from scratch and find out what will appeal to them.

The mass media have caught on to the changes in men's attitude to health perhaps more quickly than health professionals. The rapid proliferation of men's magazines, some with a high health content, bears testament to the power of accurate targeting. Although they may only be reaching certain sections of the male population, these magazines work! Men pay out good money for information that is certainly available free from existing health promotion departments and government leaflets. What these magazines have done is to think carefully about what men like, and about the way information is presented. Baker (Ch. 9) suggests there are real opportunities for health workers to influence the message these magazines carry. If men's health has become a sexy media issue, then as health workers we can take advantage of that.

Self-help

Much of the stimulus for the work health services have done since the mid-1970s on women's health has come from women themselves, and self-help groups for women continue to provide an important part of the development of better health for women. Men's health self-help groups are virtually unknown. On the whole, men have simply not seen themselves as active consumers of health information and certainly not identified themselves as a group needing particular help. There are exceptions to this – notably gay and bisexual men's campaigning and lobbying work around HIV/AIDS (and to some extent sexual health), which has forced changes in Government policy and health practice. But around other health issues this hasn't happened for men.

Williams (Ch. 10) shows just how difficult sustaining a self-help support group can be. In his case, the role of the group changed, to that of advocacy and lobbying. We would have to say that the jury is still out on whether self-help is likely to be a productive route through which men's health will be improved. However, as awareness among men rises, it may prove to be the only viable option for particular groups of men who feel excluded or marginalised by mainstream health services.

Settings

As we have seen, one of the major barriers for both men and workers in the health field has been the inappropriateness of traditional health settings. Going *where men already are* is rapidly becoming the orthodoxy for those seeking innovatory approaches. Below we will briefly consider some possible settings where health work can be done with men on their own territory.

Sport

It might be thought that sport was the last place men would want to be bothered by someone peddling better health messages. And it is certainly true that when playing or watching sport, men are simply seeking to enjoy themselves and don't have a self-improvement agenda. Competitiveness is often integral to the experience of watching or playing and emotion often gets the upper hand. Workers may balk at the idea of attempting to enter the seemingly macho atmosphere of a rugby match or a football training session. Yet both Robinson (Ch. 13) and Hamilton (Ch. 22) show that sport can be a rich forum for harnessing men's interest in healthier lifestyles.

The opportunities for health workers lie not simply in the content – most men have some interest in some sport, whether as spectators or participants – but also in the fact that this is men's territory and they are likely to feel far more confident being in a sports setting than they would at a GP's surgery or health clinic or a school PHSE lesson. The direct and practical link between diet, fitness and being better at football is used by CEDC when it runs its fitness campaign for young footballers. Robinson shows that a lot of thought needs to go into the organisation of such schemes, but that a specific message with an obvious pay-off is attractive to men.

The workplace

The workplace has increasingly been used as a setting in which to engage men on all sorts of health issues. Again it might be thought initially that men would resent health workers invading their territory by bringing health messages to work. But in practice this does not seem to have been the case. Certainly there are practical difficulties for health workers in negotiating access, and finding appropriate formats for different types of workplace and different groups of men. However, it seems that men are often more willing to attend a health lecture, discussion group or checkup if they can do so with friends or workmates. There is sometimes an increased motivation to use what is offered because it is seen by both workers and managers as being 'good for business' – in other words improving workers' health improves performance and reduces absenteeism. Men can be reached during lunchtimes, removing the necessity for them to ask for time off work. And finally, the men are in a known environment, seeing a health worker more on their terms than the other way round.

Twardzicki and Roche's work with construction workers on skin cancer (Ch. 16) is a good example of the careful preparation needed to ensure that workplace health education is meaningful and used positively. Clearly there are dangers of tokenism or manipulation from management, or hostility from the workforce if the formats used are inappropriate. However, the obvious practical application of the health message about skin cancer and the cooperative methods used meant that in the case described, health messages were taken on board by a group of men who would probably not otherwise have accessed them.

Prison

Prisons provide another alternative setting for health work – though not the most obvious one. Although the male prison population is likely to be less healthy than men 'on the outside', the quality of healthcare prisons is very variable. Overcrowding and violence combined with a lack of resources for education make it a difficult setting in which to carry out health education or provide adequate services. On the other hand it has some of the same advantages which apply to other nontraditional settings, most notably, a 'captive' audience. These are men who have time to consider this kind of issue, and probably a high degree of motivation to maintain their health and review the relationships they have in the outside world. However, as Evans shows (Ch. 17), there is much work still to be done if male prisoners are to be reached effectively with health messages and services.

Different groups of men

It is critically important that in our enthusiasm to improve men's health status and bring them in from the margins, we remember that they are not a homogenous group. Any strategic approach to men's health needs to take into account the differences between men, as well as the similarities. This means that everything we have discussed above in relation to men as a general group – that there are internal barriers for men themselves, that workers have their own barriers and that opportunities do exist once we have assessed need – must also be considered for men as members of distinct groups. Below we examine just a few of these.

Young men

The general barriers that exist for adult men in relation to accessing health services tend to be amplified for younger men. Service providers are not only unsure of what younger men want, but they are often frightened of them too. Groups of young men attending family planning clinics, for example, can be seen as 'trouble' rather than clients. And sometimes their behaviour, because of their unfamiliarity with service provision, makes them cause the expected 'trouble'. Studies have shown that young men lack confidence in the trustworthiness and confidentiality of health services. Although at school young men represent a captive audience for health educators the same lack of confidence and assumptions about lack of interest can pervade this work as it does with adult men. A vicious circle often operates here, with health workers expecting problems from young men and young men playing into this.

A big advantage we have in our work with young men is that we often have access to groups of them either through school or youth settings. Massaro (Ch. 19) makes a sound case for targeted work (in this case on sex education) with groups of young men. In particular he argues that health educators and others must seek to understand how conditioning forms their health beliefs and behaviours. Once armed with this knowledge workers can set about designing resources (see Brown Ch. 7) and methods that appeal to them.

Providers of health services will have a harder job to make them more 'young men-friendly'. Yet even here there are opportunities if time is taken to consult and find new ways of making services known to younger men. Most want to talk about health and want somewhere to go when they have a problem. Catching them young will help create a healthier adult male population.

Black men

Black men and others from ethnic minorities may experience an added layer of marginalisation from mainstream health services because of the effects of racism. Health services may well be perceived as unresponsive and, in the case of mental health, as distinctly unsympathetic or even hostile. For white workers the lack of knowledge and confidence about working with men generally may be amplified in the case of black men. As Bhavsar argues (Ch. 18) health professionals need not only to consider the different cultural beliefs and behaviours of other communities, but also the particular effect of black masculinity on attitudes to health. There is a growing recognition, confirmed by statistics, that targeting particular ethnic and racial groups is important. Work has been developed around Asian men and coronary heart disease and smoking, for example.

To break down the distance between black men and health services a re-evaluation of perspective is first needed. This can be achieved by finding out what these men need. This needs to be done for each distinct cultural group worked with. Bhavsar also suggests that, because of the distance between black men and services and the suspicion that exists, developing successful work relies on workers stepping outside orthodox approaches. This may mean a willingness to work to a broader brief than is traditionally seen in health work. As a consequence it is important that health workers build multidisciplinary strategies which can deal with the wider social issues underlying poor health.

Gay men

As has been mentioned above gay and bisexual men appear to be the exception to the rule that men are poor users of health services and unreached by health education messages. The work done on HIV/AIDS and to some extent sexual health has been among the most experimental and challenging for health services and educators. Much of this work has been done by gay men on their own initiative, but health workers have responded. However, as Hart and Flowers have shown (Ch. 20), this pioneering work reaching a marginalised group of men about a life-threatening illness has overshadowed more general health issues. The result is that gay and bisexual men's general health tends to be as little considered as the general male population's by health workers. Gay men are, after all, men and many of the factors influencing health beliefs and behaviours illustrated in Part 1 are also true for them.

Hart and Flowers suggest that the identification of gay men by health workers with *sexual* health issues does them no favours in terms of their general health needs. The challenge for workers is to step outside of stereotypes and assumptions about gay men's general health, as they have already done about their sexual health. The path to this is of course similar to work with other groups of men. Thorough needs analysis leads to better understanding and practice. The advantage workers have is that gay men have shown themselves to be health literate in terms of sexual health, and to be willing to be active consumers of health information, advice and services. The potential for transferring this interest to general health is good.

Hard-to-reach men

Another way of classifying men is to consider them in terms of their distance from services and health messages. For a long time all men were considered to be hard to reach and this underpinned the lack of development of the work. We have emphasised throughout this book the need to break down this stereotype and, whilst acknowledging the barriers, to focus on the bridges that can be built. The recent social changes described in Part 1 suggest that men can no longer easily be lumped together as totally inaccessible to health workers. Careful examination of need, reviewing of stereotypes and acknowledgement of how social changes already affect men's lives should show us that men exist on a continuum of closeness and distance to health services and messages. This means that we can subdivide men in terms of their position on this continuum and design our approach to them accordingly.

Hoare and Walsh (Ch. 6) give us a useful example of this in their classification of men as opportunistic, passive or prepared. This is a much more sophisticated approach than simply labelling men as being hard or very hard (!) to reach. It builds in an understanding of *why* men act the way they do (in this case in relation to contraception) and so enables more focused interventions to be developed. This way of looking at men's health beliefs and behaviours could be applied to many other health issues. It allows for realistic outcomes to be set for different men in different situations on different issues.

Conditions

Another way of approaching health work with men is to focus on different health conditions, e.g. coronary heart disease, testicular cancer, contraception. In the past this focus on specific conditions has meant that men have been viewed as the same as 'everybody else'. In other words an understanding of the impact of masculinity and men's conditioning on health beliefs and behaviours has been left out. Whether the condition is specific to men, or more general but affecting men, the lack of a male perspective means that we have failed to adequately address the preventable risk behaviour of men or design services which they are happy to use.

On the other hand a condition-based view can be the most accessible entry point for many men. If holistic thinking about health is still some way off for many men, then a more pragmatic, tightly focused approach can still be successful if we include an understanding of the specific issues likely to arise for men. Several of the contributors to this book start from this perspective. Both Hamilton's (Ch. 21) and Williams' (Ch. 10) work on raising awareness of testicular cancer are good examples of how a single issue can really reach men and health workers. This way of working has simple aims, provides clear outcomes and is accessible to groups of men who would not otherwise be thinking about their health. Wilkins' (Ch. 13) work on weight loss, and MacKenzie's (Ch. 22) on suicide also illustrate the benefits of restricting our agenda. Men understand what we are trying to do, other professions can see where they might contribute, and policy makers and managers can see the work meeting achievable targets.

Conclusion

In this chapter we have tried to illustrate the opportunities that exist for carrying out health work with men. Certainly barriers exist – amongst men, amongst workers and within polices and structures. However, what clearly emerges from the research and the practice we have reviewed and highlighted is that many men are motivated to better their health and that many health workers and others are succeeding in breaking through the barriers. Whilst the current policy context still has to be clarified in practice, practitioners and strategists have a better chance than ever before to ensure that men are given the healthcare they need and are seen as a legitimate audience for health messages.

Appendix 1
Further reading and resources

Introduction

This appendix contains items that we believe will be useful for those engaged in health promotion and education. There are not many books or resources directed at practice itself, and what is available is often focused on sexual health. We do not include medical texts here, except where we feel these would be of direct use to practitioners or policy makers.

For further reading and resources on men's health the reader is directed to the Health Promotion Information Centre (HPIC) at the Health Education Authority. Details of other general resources on working with men are available from Working With Men, 320 Commercial Way, London SE15 1QN.

Books

Davidson N, Lloyd T (eds) 1999 Health related resources for men. Health Education Authority, London

This book reviews all the currently available videos, packs, books, games and manuals which could be used by professionals in health related work with men and boys. It will be updated regularly on the HEA's website.

Adult men

Calman K, 1993 On the state of the public health – 1992. HMSO, London

The annual report for 1992 on the state of the nation's health which initiated much of the early interest in men's health.

Drever F, Whitehead M (eds) 1997 Health inequalities. Office for national statistics, HMSO, London

Sabo D, Gordon D F 1995 Men's health and illness. Sage, London

Academic but useful background on health and masculinity.

Young men

Lloyd T 1997 Let's get changed lads. Working With Men, London

Although not directly about health, this contains useful background on rationale and approaches to work with young men.

Blake S, Laxton J 1998 Strides – a practical guide to sex and relationships education with young men. Family Planning Association, London

Designed in participation with young men, this manual offers guidance on preparing and supporting sex education work with boys. The bulk of the book is devoted to exercises and games.

Davidson N 1997 Boys will be …? Sex education and young men. Working With Men, London

Looks at the impact of masculinity on learning to be sexual. Contains exercises for work with young men and a description of seven sex education sessions.

Lenderyou G, Ray C (eds) 1997 Let's hear it for the boys. Sex Education Forum, London.

Contains a review of the rationale for work with boys and chapters on working in sexual health services and schools, and running training.

Leaflets

Adult men

Sexual health matters for men. Health Education Authority 1997. *A 15-page booklet giving information and advice on sexual health.*

Young men

4 Boys: a below the belt guide to the male body. Family Planning Association 1995.

A pocket-sized colourful booklet for young men aged 13–16 which gives reassuring and factual information about physical changes and sexual development.

Young gay men talking. AVERT 1995

A booklet aimed at the 14–18 age group which is designed to help young men through the process of deciding whether they are gay or not and to help them deal with their feelings.

Videos

Safe. Working With Men 1996

This 22-minute drama reflects on a number of issues including responsibility, risk-taking, manhood and being young and black. Aimed at the 15–20 age group.

Packs and other resources

Addressing sun safety with out door workers: a workplace intervention pack. Health Education Authority 1998.

This comprehensive pack on sun safety, put together by Twardzicki and Roche (see Ch. 17), is aimed at anyone providing health information in the workplace. It contains guidance, training materials and background information.

It Takes Two: creating opportunities for clients. Sexual health, contraception and men. A training resource. Contraceptive Education Service, Health Education Authority 1998

This pack of research findings and training exercises aims to help health professionals integrate men into the 'contraceptive culture'. It offers ways of increasing effective communication between professionals and men.

Male image photopack. Working With Men 1995

52 photos of a diverse range of men in a variety of situations.

A useful general resource for helping men start discussing masculinity, roles and behaviours.

TSE practice model. Available from: Philip Harris Health Education, Gazelle Road, Weston Industrial Estate, Weston-Super-Mare, Avon BS21 9BG.

Model of scrotum and testicles for teaching men testicular self-examination.

Background statistical information

Bradford N 1995 Men's health matters. Vermillion, London

A comprehensive guide to men's health, from beer guts and baldness through to sexual difficulties.

Carroll S 1994 The Which? guide to men's health. Consumers' Association, London

All the facts on men's physical, sexual and emotional health.

Davidson N 1995 Vitality and virility – a guide to sexual health for mid-life men. Ace Books, London

Contains sections on most sexual health issues affecting men, such as impotence and premature ejaculation.

Davidson N, Lloyd T 1995 Working with heterosexual men on sexual health. Health Education Authority, London

An audit of approaches to work with men, covering peer education, HIV, men with learning difficulties, etc.

Harrison T, Dignan K (eds) 1999 Men's health: an introduction for nurses and health professionals. Churchill Livingstone, London

Illustrates issues in the current debate around men's health and provides information on background issues.

Hazelhurst M 1993 Breaking in … Breaking out. (Social and sex education for men with learning difficulties.) Working With Men, London

Useful books linking men with learning difficulties and masculinity

Lloyd T 1996 The men's health review. Royal College of Nursing, London

Background statistics and a review of literature on men's health issues.

O' Dowd T, Jewell D 1998 Men's health. Oxford University Press, Oxford.

Contains relevant statistical information for those involved in primary care.

Appendix 2

Alive and Kicking task sheets

This appendix contains two examples of the task sheets used in the *Alive and Kicking* project described in Chapter 13. They are:

- task sheet six–diet
- task sheet eight–mental health.

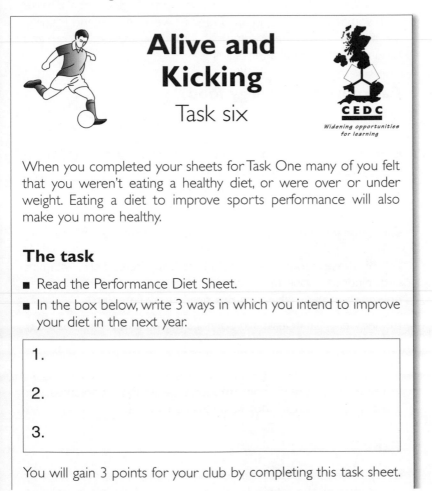

Alive and Kicking

Task six

CEDC

Widening opportunities for learning

When you completed your sheets for Task One many of you felt that you weren't eating a healthy diet, or were over or under weight. Eating a diet to improve sports performance will also make you more healthy.

The task

- Read the Performance Diet Sheet.
- In the box below, write 3 ways in which you intend to improve your diet in the next year.

1.

2.

3.

You will gain 3 points for your club by completing this task sheet.

Diet sheet

Eating for improved football performance has to be maintained: attention must be paid to eating habits for 365 days of the year, not just on match days. You need a good balance of food, which will supply you with the fuel that your body needs for high-grade performance.

Here are some pointers to success:

Organise yourself

Remember that you must refuel, so don't neglect meals: make sure you fit your eating in around your work, leisure and training. When you train in the evening, eat something around 3–4 pm and have your main meal after training.

Eat more low-energy food

Eat more:

- fresh or frozen vegetables (particularly root varieties and green leafy vegetables), potatoes;
- fresh and dried fruit (particularly citrus fruits);
- cereals (wholemeal pasta, brown rice, muesli, etc.);
- nuts, beans and pulses (peas, all types of beans, lentils, etc.).

All of these foods are high in carbohydrate, fibre, vitamins and minerals in one tasty package. They are also relatively low in energy, so in themselves are not significantly fattening.

Remember – eat at least five portions of fruit and vegetables a day.

Bread

Increase your bread consumption (preferably wholemeal or granary) but take care not to add lashings of fat.

Fat

- Try to reduce the overall amount of fat in your diet. Start by reducing all the visible fat (butter, oils, lard, fat on meat) and non-visible fat (milk, dairy produce, eggs, mayonnaise, sausages, paté, batter, pies and pastry) in your diet. Switch to low-fat spreads, skimmed milk and low-fat cheese.

■ Reduce your consumption of fried foods – try grilling, stir-frying or steaming.

Meat and fish

There is no need to eat large amounts of red meat. Replace high-fat meats (lamb, beef, pork and duck) with lean or white meats (chicken, turkey, etc.). Similarly replace oily fish (mackerel, tuna, etc.) with white fish. Or reduce your meat eating and fill up on bread and pasta.

Fluid intake

Ensure that you maintain a high fluid intake by drinking plenty of water and fresh fruit juice (high in minerals) as part of your normal diet. Always take care not to become dehydrated before or during any training session or match. Organise yourself so that you can take small amounts of fluid regularly. Be careful of alcohol – don't try to play or train on a hangover.

Breakfast

Start the day with a breakfast that is high in complex carbo-hydrates – muesli or whole-grain cereals are much better than sweetened cereal products. Skimmed milk, fresh fruit juice, tea or coffee will all provide liquid without excessive fat. If you miss breakfast because of jogging or training (!), use handy high-carbo-hydrate muesli or fruit and nut bars.

Snacks

Try taking smaller and more frequent meals. Mid-morning or after-noon snacks can help, particularly when training in the early evening, but don't start an eating habit which may eventually lead to five or six meals a day!

If you follow this eating guide to increasing your football perfor-mance, you will also improve your general health.

Alive and Kicking

Task Eight

CEDC

Widening opportunities for learning

Name ....

Club ....

Spotting the Signs

One of the most important points to remember is that a healthy mind is as important as a healthy body. We all feel depressed, anxious or confused sometimes, particularly after a distressing life event such as losing someone you love. Most of us cope with these feelings with time, especially if we have the support of family and friends. However, it is important to know how to spot the signs of more deep-seated stress or depression in yourself or those close to you. We enclose a beer mat to help you spot the signs that further support might be needed.

The task

You will find attached a questionnaire called 'Mind Games'. Complete the questionnaire 'Are you a winner or a loser?' **honestly**. In the box below, write your score.

Score　　　　　　　　　(you obtain 3 points for entering your score)

If you are a type A personality also write down two things you will do to manage your 'A' personality.

Are you a winner or a loser?

Cut out the psycho-babble and get your mind fit for the game ahead with our workout. Increase your mental flexibility with our 'suppling exercises' before or after a game or any time you need to wind down or focus your energies.

Try to work out and find out if you've won or lost the game in your head even before you've put your kit on.

6. When you're talking to your mates do you:

   a. wave your arms about a lot □ (1)

   b. accentuate key words □ (2)

   c. speak faster as you near the end of what you have to say □ (3)

   d. say very little? □ (4)

2. If you got to a training session an hour early because someone told you the wrong time, would you:

   a. resent wasting time and get started on a really good workout □ (3)

   b. feel frustrated and go down the pub □ (2)

   c. get angry and plan what you are going to say when the rest arrive □ (1)

   d. get a newspaper and enjoy a free hour? □ (4)

3. When you look through the results, do you:

   a. just read the scorelines if you get the time □ (1)

   b. relax and read the full match report □ (4)

   c. half-read the scorelines while you're doing something else □ (2)

   d. ask your mates about the results later? □ (3)

4. If you play an away match in a part of the country you've not been to before, do you:

   a. feel you don't have time to notice anything other than the game □ (1)

   b. have a look around the ground □ (2)

   c. look forward to seeing what the area looks like □ (3)

   d. plan to stop over and get out and about? □ (4)

5. In training, do you:
   a. rate your abilities against everyone else ☐ (2)
   b. patiently watch new players learn the ropes ☐ (4)
   c. feel frustrated that you're not progressing
      quickly enough ☐ (3)
   d. feel compelled to challenge the most
      competitive players? ☐ (1)

6. When road directions to the away match are being explained,
   do you:
   a. listen carefully ☐ (4)
   b. grind your teeth, tap your foot or develop a
      nervous tic ☐ (1)
   c. want to chip in with a better route ☐ (3)
   d. feel impatient and keep saying 'Yes' or 'Uh huh?' ☐ (2)

How did you score?

6–15 Points:

You're trying hard, in fact you're working hard at being the best. You
are competitive to the point of aggression, which can get you into
difficulties with the team. You can be a liability on the pitch because
of your temper. You are very aware of time and dislike being kept
waiting. Winning and achievement are important to you and you
never admit being tired or not being able to cope. Relaxation is
something other people do. You are a classic type A personality.

15–24 Points:

Life is full of opportunities. You know how to make the most of
every situation and stay calm. You're not hurried or bothered by
other people trying to get one over on you. You know lots about
football because you take the time to read up and listen to other
people. Others in the team rely on you. You are a classic type B
personality.

Why type A personality people are the losers

Research studies have shown that type A behaviour have double
the risk of heart disease and other stress-related conditions. They
may be high achievers but the excessive discharge of stress
hormones can lead to problems on and off the pitch. The good

news is that type As can learn to manage their behaviour without impairing performance.

If you are a type A personality try our workout below and maximise your performance.

Managing type A behaviour

Identify your type A behaviour on a checklist and then make deliberate attempts to 'go against the grain' and alter that behaviour by the following methods:

1 Practise being a good listener. Search out somebody who talks slowly and deliberately. Have a slow conversation. Try to hold back from making yourself the centre of attention by asking yourself 'Do I really have anything important to say?'.

2 Be aware of your obsessional time-directed lifestyle and try to slow down. Deliberately walk or eat slowly, setting aside a specified time period when you have to stay at the dinner table. Penalise yourself if you catch yourself speeding up in the car or jumping a red light.

3 Build into your daily and weekly timetable stress-free 'breathing spaces', when you deliberately try to relax. This might be a five-minute period when you carry out a muscle relaxation exercise, a walk in the park at lunchtime, or a break when you read the newspaper.

4 As part of an effort to broaden yourself and reduce obsessional time-directed behaviour, deliberately develop leisure activities and hobbies, for example, sailing, gardening or walking. Commit yourself fully to these activities.

5 Try to adopt a more positive approach to expressing yourself and how you feel. Take time to thank others and show appreciation when somebody has done something for you. Talk to others about how you are feeling – ventilate feelings rather than bottling them up.

6 Take time out to assess the cause of your type A behaviour – hurry, sickness, hostility and competitiveness. Ask yourself, 'What am I trying to prove?'. Pay particular attention to looking at things you value most in life. How are they related to this type A behaviour? Does your idealism and striving improve or diminish the quality of your life?

Index